THE OFFICIAL PATIENT'S SOURCEBOOK

on

POLYCYSTIC KIDNEY DISEASE

JAMES N. PARKER, M.D.
AND PHILIP M. PARKER, PH.D., EDITORS

ICON Health Publications
ICON Group International, Inc.
4370 La Jolla Village Drive, 4th Floor
San Diego, CA 92122 USA

Copyright ©2002 by ICON Group International, Inc.

Printed in the United States of America.

Last digit indicates print number: 10 9 8 7 6 4 5 3 2 1

Publisher, Health Care: Tiffany LaRochelle
Editor(s): James Parker, M.D., Philip Parker, Ph.D.

Publisher's note: The ideas, procedures, and suggestions contained in this book are not intended as a substitute for consultation with your physician. All matters regarding your health require medical supervision. As new medical or scientific information becomes available from academic and clinical research, recommended treatments and drug therapies may undergo changes. The authors, editors, and publisher have attempted to make the information in this book up to date and accurate in accord with accepted standards at the time of publication. The authors, editors, and publisher are not responsible for errors or omissions or for consequences from application of the book, and make no warranty, expressed or implied, in regard to the contents of this book. Any practice described in this book should be applied by the reader in accordance with professional standards of care used in regard to the unique circumstances that may apply in each situation, in close consultation with a qualified physician. The reader is advised to always check product information (package inserts) for changes and new information regarding dose and contraindications before taking any drug or pharmacological product. Caution is especially urged when using new or infrequently ordered drugs, herbal remedies, vitamins and supplements, alternative therapies, complementary therapies and medicines, and integrative medical treatments.

Cataloging-in-Publication Data

Parker, James N., 1961-
Parker, Philip M., 1960-

    The Official Patient's Sourcebook on Polycystic Kidney Disease: A Revised and Updated Directory for the Internet Age/James N. Parker and Philip M. Parker, editors
         p.   cm.
    Includes bibliographical references, glossary and index.
    ISBN: 0-597-83227-7
    1. Polycystic Kidney Disease-Popular works.   I. Title.

Disclaimer

This publication is not intended to be used for the diagnosis or treatment of a health problem or as a substitute for consultation with licensed medical professionals. It is sold with the understanding that the publisher, editors, and authors are not engaging in the rendering of medical, psychological, financial, legal, or other professional services.

References to any entity, product, service, or source of information that may be contained in this publication should not be considered an endorsement, either direct or implied, by the publisher, editors or authors. ICON Group International, Inc., the editors, or the authors are not responsible for the content of any Web pages nor publications referenced in this publication.

Copyright Notice

Dedication

To the healthcare professionals dedicating their time and efforts to the study of polycystic kidney disease.

Acknowledgements

The collective knowledge generated from academic and applied research summarized in various references has been critical in the creation of this sourcebook which is best viewed as a comprehensive compilation and collection of information prepared by various official agencies which directly or indirectly are dedicated to polycystic kidney disease. All of the *Official Patient's Sourcebooks* draw from various agencies and institutions associated with the United States Department of Health and Human Services, and in particular, the Office of the Secretary of Health and Human Services (OS), the Administration for Children and Families (ACF), the Administration on Aging (AOA), the Agency for Healthcare Research and Quality (AHRQ), the Agency for Toxic Substances and Disease Registry (ATSDR), the Centers for Disease Control and Prevention (CDC), the Food and Drug Administration (FDA), the Healthcare Financing Administration (HCFA), the Health Resources and Services Administration (HRSA), the Indian Health Service (IHS), the institutions of the National Institutes of Health (NIH), the Program Support Center (PSC), and the Substance Abuse and Mental Health Services Administration (SAMHSA). In addition to these sources, information gathered from the National Library of Medicine, the United States Patent Office, the European Union, and their related organizations has been invaluable in the creation of this sourcebook. Some of the work represented was financially supported by the Research and Development Committee at INSEAD. This support is gratefully acknowledged. Finally, special thanks are owed to Tiffany LaRochelle for her excellent editorial support.

About the Editors

James N. Parker, M.D.

Dr. James N. Parker received his Bachelor of Science degree in Psychobiology from the University of California, Riverside and his M.D. from the University of California, San Diego. In addition to authoring numerous research publications, he has lectured at various academic institutions. Dr. Parker is the medical editor for the *Official Patient's Sourcebook* series published by ICON Health Publications.

Philip M. Parker, Ph.D.

Philip M. Parker is the Eli Lilly Chair Professor of Innovation, Business and Society at INSEAD (Fontainebleau, France and Singapore). Dr. Parker has also been Professor at the University of California, San Diego and has taught courses at Harvard University, the Hong Kong University of Science and Technology, the Massachusetts Institute of Technology, Stanford University, and UCLA. Dr. Parker is the associate editor for the *Official Patient's Sourcebook* series published by ICON Health Publications.

About ICON Health Publications

In addition to polycystic kidney disease, *Official Patient's Sourcebooks* are available for the following related topics:

- The Official Patient's Sourcebook on Childhood Nephrotic Syndrome
- The Official Patient's Sourcebook on Cystocele
- The Official Patient's Sourcebook on Glomerular Disease
- The Official Patient's Sourcebook on Goodpasture Syndrome
- The Official Patient's Sourcebook on Hematuria
- The Official Patient's Sourcebook on Hemochromatosis
- The Official Patient's Sourcebook on Immune Thrombocytopenic Purpura
- The Official Patient's Sourcebook on Impotence
- The Official Patient's Sourcebook on Interstitial Cystitis
- The Official Patient's Sourcebook on Kidney Failure
- The Official Patient's Sourcebook on Kidney Stones
- The Official Patient's Sourcebook on Lupus Nephritis
- The Official Patient's Sourcebook on Nephrotic Syndrome
- The Official Patient's Sourcebook on Peyronie
- The Official Patient's Sourcebook on Prostate Enlargement
- The Official Patient's Sourcebook on Prostatitis
- The Official Patient's Sourcebook on Proteinuria
- The Official Patient's Sourcebook on Pyelonephritis
- The Official Patient's Sourcebook on Renal Osteodystrophy
- The Official Patient's Sourcebook on Renal Tubular Acidosis
- The Official Patient's Sourcebook on Simple Kidney Cysts
- The Official Patient's Sourcebook on Urinary Incontinence
- The Official Patient's Sourcebook on Urinary Incontinence for Women
- The Official Patient's Sourcebook on Urinary Tract Infection in Children
- The Official Patient's Sourcebook on Urinary Tract Infections in Adults
- The Official Patient's Sourcebook on Vasectomy
- The Official Patient's Sourcebook on Vesicoureteral Reflux

To discover more about ICON Health Publications, simply check with your preferred online booksellers, including Barnes & Noble.com and Amazon.com which currently carry all of our titles. Or, feel free to contact us directly for bulk purchases or institutional discounts:

ICON Group International, Inc.
4370 La Jolla Village Drive, Fourth Floor
San Diego, CA 92122 USA
Fax: 858-546-4341
Web site: **www.icongrouponline.com/health**

Table of Contents

INTRODUCTION..1
    Overview 1
    Organization 3
    Scope 3
    Moving Forward 5

PART I: THE ESSENTIALS...7

  CHAPTER 1. THE ESSENTIALS ON POLYCYSTIC KIDNEY DISEASE: GUIDELINES.....9
    Overview 9
    What Is Polycystic Kidney Disease? 11
    What Is Autosomal Dominant PKD 12
    What Are the Symptoms of Autosomal Dominant PKD? 12
    How Is Autosomal Dominant PKD Diagnosed? 13
    How Is Autosomal Dominant PKD Treated? 14
    What Is Autosomal Recessive PKD? 15
    What Are the Symptoms of Autosomal Recessive PKD? 15
    How Is Autosomal Recessive PKD Diagnosed? 16
    How Is Autosomal Recessive PKD Treated? 16
    Genetic Diseases...16
    What Is Acquired Cystic Kidney Disease 17
    How Is ACKD Diagnosed?..17
    How Is ACKD Treated? 17
    The Search for PKD Genes 17
    Points to Remember..18
    Additional Resources 19
    More Guideline Sources 20
    Vocabulary Builder...24
  CHAPTER 2. SEEKING GUIDANCE..27
    Overview 27
    Associations and Polycystic Kidney Disease...27
    Finding More Associations 30
    Finding Doctors 32
    Finding a Urologist 33
    Selecting Your Doctor 33
    Working with Your Doctor...34
    Broader Health-Related Resources...35
    Vocabulary Builder...36

PART II: ADDITIONAL RESOURCES AND ADVANCED MATERIAL...................37

  CHAPTER 3. STUDIES ON POLYCYSTIC KIDNEY DISEASE..39
    Overview 39
    The Combined Health Information Database 39
    Federally-Funded Research on Polycystic Kidney Disease 48
    E-Journals: PubMed Central 64
    The National Library of Medicine: PubMed 66
    Vocabulary Builder...67
  CHAPTER 4. PATENTS ON POLYCYSTIC KIDNEY DISEASE 73
    Overview 73
    Patents on Polycystic Kidney Disease 74
    Patent Applications on Polycystic Kidney Disease 77
    Keeping Current 78

CHAPTER 5. BOOKS ON POLYCYSTIC KIDNEY DISEASE 79
    Overview 79
    Book Summaries: Federal Agencies 79
    Book Summaries: Online Booksellers 81
    The National Library of Medicine Book Index 81
    Chapters on Polycystic Kidney Disease 83
    Directories...87
    General Home References 88
    Vocabulary Builder 89
CHAPTER 6. MULTIMEDIA ON POLYCYSTIC KIDNEY DISEASE 91
    Overview 91
    Video Recordings...91
    Bibliography: Multimedia on Polycystic Kidney Disease 92
    Vocabulary Builder...93
CHAPTER 7. PERIODICALS AND NEWS ON POLYCYSTIC KIDNEY DISEASE............95
    Overview 95
    News Services & Press Releases 95
    Newsletter Articles 98
    Academic Periodicals covering Polycystic Kidney Disease..101
    Vocabulary Builder...102
CHAPTER 8. PHYSICIAN GUIDELINES AND DATABASES...103
    Overview 103
    NIH Guidelines..103
    NIH Databases...104
    Other Commercial Databases...109
    The Genome Project and Polycystic Kidney Disease...110
    Specialized References 114
    Vocabulary Builder...115
CHAPTER 9. DISSERTATIONS ON POLYCYSTIC KIDNEY DISEASE 117
    Overview 117
    Dissertations on Polycystic Kidney Disease 117
    Keeping Current 118
    Vocabulary Builder...118

PART III. APPENDICES 119

APPENDIX A. RESEARCHING YOUR MEDICATIONS...121
    Overview 121
    Your Medications: The Basics...122
    Learning More about Your Medications..124
    Commercial Databases 125
    Contraindications and Interactions (Hidden Dangers) 126
    A Final Warning..127
    General References..128
    Vocabulary Builder...129
APPENDIX B. RESEARCHING ALTERNATIVE MEDICINE..131
    Overview 131
    What Is CAM? 131
    What Are the Domains of Alternative Medicine? 132
    Can Alternatives Affect My Treatment? 135
    Finding CAM References on Polycystic Kidney Disease 136
    Additional Web Resources 141
    General References..142
    Vocabulary Builder...143
APPENDIX C. RESEARCHING NUTRITION..145

Overview *145*
Food and Nutrition: General Principles *145*
Finding Studies on Polycystic Kidney Disease *150*
Federal Resources on Nutrition *154*
Additional Web Resources *155*
Vocabulary Builder *155*
APPENDIX D. FINDING MEDICAL LIBRARIES *157*
Overview *157*
Preparation *157*
Finding a Local Medical Library *158*
Medical Libraries Open to the Public *158*
APPENDIX E. YOUR RIGHTS AND INSURANCE *165*
Overview *165*
Your Rights as a Patient *165*
Patient Responsibilities *169*
Choosing an Insurance Plan *170*
Medicare and Medicaid *173*
NORD's Medication Assistance Programs *176*
Additional Resources *176*
APPENDIX F. ANEMIA IN KIDNEY DISEASE *179*
Overview *179*
Laboratory Tests *180*
When Anemia Begins *180*
Diagnosis *181*
Treatment *181*
Other Causes of Anemia *182*
Hope through Research *183*
For More Information *184*

ONLINE GLOSSARIES **187**
Online Dictionary Directories *194*

POLYCYSTIC KIDNEY DISEASE GLOSSARY **195**
General Dictionaries and Glossaries *207*

INDEX...**209**

INTRODUCTION

Overview

Dr. C. Everett Koop, former U.S. Surgeon General, once said, "The best prescription is knowledge."[1] The Agency for Healthcare Research and Quality (AHRQ) of the National Institutes of Health (NIH) echoes this view and recommends that every patient incorporate education into the treatment process. According to the AHRQ:

> Finding out more about your condition is a good place to start. By contacting groups that support your condition, visiting your local library, and searching on the Internet, you can find good information to help guide your treatment decisions. Some information may be hard to find — especially if you don't know where to look.[2]

As the AHRQ mentions, finding the right information is not an obvious task. Though many physicians and public officials had thought that the emergence of the Internet would do much to assist patients in obtaining reliable information, in March 2001 the National Institutes of Health issued the following warning:

> The number of Web sites offering health-related resources grows every day. Many sites provide valuable information, while others may have information that is unreliable or misleading.[3]

---

[1] Quotation from **http://www.drkoop.com**.

[2] The Agency for Healthcare Research and Quality (AHRQ):
http://www.ahcpr.gov/consumer/diaginfo.htm.

[3] From the NIH, National Cancer Institute (NCI):
http://cancertrials.nci.nih.gov/beyond/evaluating.html.

Since the late 1990s, physicians have seen a general increase in patient Internet usage rates. Patients frequently enter their doctor's offices with printed Web pages of home remedies in the guise of latest medical research. This scenario is so common that doctors often spend more time dispelling misleading information than guiding patients through sound therapies. *The Official Patient's Sourcebook on Polycystic Kidney Disease* has been created for patients who have decided to make education and research an integral part of the treatment process. The pages that follow will tell you where and how to look for information covering virtually all topics related to polycystic kidney disease, from the essentials to the most advanced areas of research.

The title of this book includes the word "official." This reflects the fact that the sourcebook draws from public, academic, government, and peer-reviewed research. Selected readings from various agencies are reproduced to give you some of the latest official information available to date on polycystic kidney disease.

Given patients' increasing sophistication in using the Internet, abundant references to reliable Internet-based resources are provided throughout this sourcebook. Where possible, guidance is provided on how to obtain free-of-charge, primary research results as well as more detailed information via the Internet. E-book and electronic versions of this sourcebook are fully interactive with each of the Internet sites mentioned (clicking on a hyperlink automatically opens your browser to the site indicated). Hard copy users of this sourcebook can type cited Web addresses directly into their browsers to obtain access to the corresponding sites. Since we are working with ICON Health Publications, hard copy *Sourcebooks* are frequently updated and printed on demand to ensure that the information provided is current.

In addition to extensive references accessible via the Internet, every chapter presents a "Vocabulary Builder." Many health guides offer glossaries of technical or uncommon terms in an appendix. In editing this sourcebook, we have decided to place a smaller glossary within each chapter that covers terms used in that chapter. Given the technical nature of some chapters, you may need to revisit many sections. Building one's vocabulary of medical terms in such a gradual manner has been shown to improve the learning process.

We must emphasize that no sourcebook on polycystic kidney disease should affirm that a specific diagnostic procedure or treatment discussed in a research study, patent, or doctoral dissertation is "correct" or your best option. This sourcebook is no exception. Each patient is unique. Deciding on appropriate options is always up to the patient in consultation with their physician and healthcare providers.

Organization

This sourcebook is organized into three parts. Part I explores basic techniques to researching polycystic kidney disease (e.g. finding guidelines on diagnosis, treatments, and prognosis), followed by a number of topics, including information on how to get in touch with organizations, associations, or other patient networks dedicated to polycystic kidney disease. It also gives you sources of information that can help you find a doctor in your local area specializing in treating polycystic kidney disease. Collectively, the material presented in Part I is a complete primer on basic research topics for patients with polycystic kidney disease.

Part II moves on to advanced research dedicated to polycystic kidney disease. Part II is intended for those willing to invest many hours of hard work and study. It is here that we direct you to the latest scientific and applied research on polycystic kidney disease. When possible, contact names, links via the Internet, and summaries are provided. It is in Part II where the vocabulary process becomes important as authors publishing advanced research frequently use highly specialized language. In general, every attempt is made to recommend "free-to-use" options.

Part III provides appendices of useful background reading for all patients with polycystic kidney disease or related disorders. The appendices are dedicated to more pragmatic issues faced by many patients with polycystic kidney disease. Accessing materials via medical libraries may be the only option for some readers, so a guide is provided for finding local medical libraries which are open to the public. Part III, therefore, focuses on advice that goes beyond the biological and scientific issues facing patients with polycystic kidney disease.

Scope

While this sourcebook covers polycystic kidney disease, your doctor, research publications, and specialists may refer to your condition using a variety of terms. Therefore, you should understand that polycystic kidney disease is often considered a synonym or a condition closely related to the following:

- Autosomal Dominant Polycystic Kidney Disease
- Autosomal Dominant Polycystic Kidney Disease (adpkd)
- Cystic Disease of the Renal Medulla
- Cysts - Kidneys
- Cysts of the Renal Medulla, Congenital
- Familial Juvenile Nephrophthisis
- Kidney - Polycystic
- Polycystic Kidney Disease, Medullary Type
- Polycystic Renal Diseases
- Senior-loken Syndrome

In addition to synonyms and related conditions, physicians may refer to polycystic kidney disease using certain coding systems. The International Classification of Diseases, 9th Revision, Clinical Modification (ICD-9-CM) is the most commonly used system of classification for the world's illnesses. Your physician may use this coding system as an administrative or tracking tool. The following classification is commonly used for polycystic kidney disease:[4]

- 753.1 polycystic kidney, unspecified type
- 753.12 polycystic kidney, unspecified type
- 753.13 polycystic kidney, autosomal dominant
- 753.13 polycystic kidney, autsomal dominant
- 753.14 polycystic kidney, autosomal recessive

For the purposes of this sourcebook, we have attempted to be as inclusive as possible, looking for official information for all of the synonyms relevant to polycystic kidney disease. You may find it useful to refer to synonyms when accessing databases or interacting with healthcare professionals and medical librarians.

---

[4] This list is based on the official version of the World Health Organization's 9th Revision, International Classification of Diseases (ICD-9). According to the National Technical Information Service, "ICD-9CM extensions, interpretations, modifications, addenda, or errata other than those approved by the U.S. Public Health Service and the Health Care Financing Administration are not to be considered official and should not be utilized. Continuous maintenance of the ICD-9-CM is the responsibility of the federal government."

Moving Forward

Since the 1980s, the world has seen a proliferation of healthcare guides covering most illnesses. Some are written by patients or their family members. These generally take a layperson's approach to understanding and coping with an illness or disorder. They can be uplifting, encouraging, and highly supportive. Other guides are authored by physicians or other healthcare providers who have a more clinical outlook. Each of these two styles of guide has its purpose and can be quite useful.

As editors, we have chosen a third route. We have chosen to expose you to as many sources of official and peer-reviewed information as practical, for the purpose of educating you about basic and advanced knowledge as recognized by medical science today. You can think of this sourcebook as your personal Internet age reference librarian.

Why "Internet age"? All too often, patients diagnosed with polycystic kidney disease will log on to the Internet, type words into a search engine, and receive several Web site listings which are mostly irrelevant or redundant. These patients are left to wonder where the relevant information is, and how to obtain it. Since only the smallest fraction of information dealing with polycystic kidney disease is even indexed in search engines, a non-systematic approach often leads to frustration and disappointment. With this sourcebook, we hope to direct you to the information you need that you would not likely find using popular Web directories. Beyond Web listings, in many cases we will reproduce brief summaries or abstracts of available reference materials. These abstracts often contain distilled information on topics of discussion.

While we focus on the more scientific aspects of polycystic kidney disease, there is, of course, the emotional side to consider. Later in the sourcebook, we provide a chapter dedicated to helping you find peer groups and associations that can provide additional support beyond research produced by medical science. We hope that the choices we have made give you the most options available in moving forward. In this way, we wish you the best in your efforts to incorporate this educational approach into your treatment plan.

The Editors

PART I: THE ESSENTIALS

ABOUT PART I

Part I has been edited to give you access to what we feel are "the essentials" on polycystic kidney disease. The essentials of a disease typically include the definition or description of the disease, a discussion of who it affects, the signs or symptoms associated with the disease, tests or diagnostic procedures that might be specific to the disease, and treatments for the disease. Your doctor or healthcare provider may have already explained the essentials of polycystic kidney disease to you or even given you a pamphlet or brochure describing polycystic kidney disease. Now you are searching for more in-depth information. As editors, we have decided, nevertheless, to include a discussion on where to find essential information that can complement what your doctor has already told you. In this section we recommend a process, not a particular Web site or reference book. The process ensures that, as you search the Web, you gain background information in such a way as to maximize your understanding.

CHAPTER 1. THE ESSENTIALS ON POLYCYSTIC KIDNEY DISEASE: GUIDELINES

Overview

Official agencies, as well as federally-funded institutions supported by national grants, frequently publish a variety of guidelines on polycystic kidney disease. These are typically called "Fact Sheets" or "Guidelines." They can take the form of a brochure, information kit, pamphlet, or flyer. Often they are only a few pages in length. The great advantage of guidelines over other sources is that they are often written with the patient in mind. Since new guidelines on polycystic kidney disease can appear at any moment and be published by a number of sources, the best approach to finding guidelines is to systematically scan the Internet-based services that post them.

The National Institutes of Health (NIH)[5]

The National Institutes of Health (NIH) is the first place to search for relatively current patient guidelines and fact sheets on polycystic kidney disease. Originally founded in 1887, the NIH is one of the world's foremost medical research centers and the federal focal point for medical research in the United States. At any given time, the NIH supports some 35,000 research grants at universities, medical schools, and other research and training institutions, both nationally and internationally. The rosters of those who have conducted research or who have received NIH support over the years include the world's most illustrious scientists and physicians. Among them are 97 scientists who have won the Nobel Prize for achievement in medicine.

---

[5] Adapted from the NIH: **http://www.nih.gov/about/NIHoverview.html**.

There is no guarantee that any one Institute will have a guideline on a specific disease, though the National Institutes of Health collectively publish over 600 guidelines for both common and rare diseases. The best way to access NIH guidelines is via the Internet. Although the NIH is organized into many different Institutes and Offices, the following is a list of key Web sites where you are most likely to find NIH clinical guidelines and publications dealing with polycystic kidney disease and associated conditions:

- Office of the Director (OD); guidelines consolidated across agencies available at **http://www.nih.gov/health/consumer/conkey.htm**

- National Library of Medicine (NLM); extensive encyclopedia (A.D.A.M., Inc.) with guidelines available at **http://www.nlm.nih.gov/medlineplus/healthtopics.html**

- National Institute of Diabetes and Digestive and Kidney Diseases (NIDDK); guidelines available at **http://www.niddk.nih.gov/health/health.htm**

Among these, the National Institute of Diabetes and Digestive and Kidney Diseases (NIDDK) is particularly noteworthy. The NIDDK's mission is to conduct and support research on many of the most serious diseases affecting public health.[6] The Institute supports much of the clinical research on the diseases of internal medicine and related subspecialty fields as well as many basic science disciplines. The NIDDK's Division of Intramural Research encompasses the broad spectrum of metabolic diseases such as diabetes, inborn errors of metabolism, endocrine disorders, mineral metabolism, digestive diseases, nutrition, urology and renal disease, and hematology. Basic research studies include biochemistry, nutrition, pathology, histochemistry, chemistry, physical, chemical, and molecular biology, pharmacology, and toxicology. NIDDK extramural research is organized into divisions of program areas:

- Division of Diabetes, Endocrinology, and Metabolic Diseases

- Division of Digestive Diseases and Nutrition

- Division of Kidney, Urologic, and Hematologic Diseases

The Division of Extramural Activities provides administrative support and overall coordination. A fifth division, the Division of Nutrition Research Coordination, coordinates government nutrition research efforts. The Institute supports basic and clinical research through investigator-initiated

---

[6] This paragraph has been adapted from the NIDDK:
http://www.niddk.nih.gov/welcome/mission.htm. "Adapted" signifies that a passage is reproduced exactly or slightly edited for this book.

grants, program project and center grants, and career development and training awards. The Institute also supports research and development projects and large-scale clinical trials through contracts. The following patient guideline was recently published by the NIDDK on polycystic kidney disease.

What Is Polycystic Kidney Disease?[7]

Polycystic kidney disease (PKD) is a genetic disorder characterized by the growth of numerous cysts in the kidneys. The cysts are filled with fluid. PKD cysts can slowly replace much of the mass of the kidneys, reducing kidney function and leading to kidney failure.

The kidneys are two organs, each about the size of a fist, located in the upper part of a person's abdomen, toward the back. The kidneys filter wastes from the blood to form urine. They also regulate amounts of certain vital substances in the body.

When PKD causes kidneys to fail--which usually happens only after many years--the patient requires dialysis or kidney transplantation. About one-half of people with the major type of PKD progress to kidney failure, i.e., end-stage renal disease (ESRD).

PKD can cause cysts in the liver and problems in other organs, such as the heart and blood vessels in the brain. These complications help doctors distinguish PKD from the usually harmless "simple" cysts that often form in the kidneys in later years of life.

In the United States, about 500,000 people have PKD, and it is the fourth leading cause of kidney failure. Medical professionals describe two major inherited forms of PKD and a noninherited form:

- Autosomal dominant PKD is the most common, inherited form. Symptoms usually develop between the ages of 30 and 40, but they can begin earlier, even in childhood. About 90 percent of all PKD cases are autosomal dominant PKD.

- Autosomal recessive PKD is a rare, inherited form. Symptoms of autosomal recessive PKD begin in the earliest months of life, even in the womb.

---

[7] Adapted from the National Institute of Diabetes and Digestive and Kidney Diseases (NIDDK): **http://www.niddk.nih.gov/health/kidney/pubs/polycyst/polycyst.htm**.

- Acquired cystic kidney disease (ACKD) develops in association with long-term kidney problems, especially in patients who have kidney failure and who have been on dialysis for a long time. Therefore it tends to occur in later years of life. It is not an inherited form of PKD.

What Is Autosomal Dominant PKD

Autosomal dominant PKD is one of the most common inherited disorders. The phrase "autosomal dominant" means that if one parent has the disease, there is a 50-percent chance that the disease will pass to a child. At least one parent must have the disease for a child to inherit it. Either the mother or father can pass it along, but new mutations may account for one-fourth of new cases. In some rare cases, the cause of autosomal dominant PKD occurs spontaneously in the child soon after conception--in these cases the parents are not the source of this disease.

Many people with autosomal dominant PKD live for decades without developing symptoms. For this reason, autosomal dominant PKD is often called "adult polycystic kidney disease." Yet, in some cases, cysts may form earlier, even in the first years of life.

The disease is thought to occur equally in men and women and equally in people of all races. However, some studies suggest that it occurs more often in whites than in blacks and more often in females than in males. High blood pressure occurs early in the disease, often before cysts appear.

The cysts grow out of nephrons, the tiny filtering units inside the kidneys. The cysts eventually separate from the nephrons and continue to enlarge. The kidneys enlarge along with the cysts (which can number in the thousands), while retaining roughly their kidney shape. In fully developed PKD, a cyst-filled kidney can weigh as much as 22 pounds.

What Are the Symptoms of Autosomal Dominant PKD?

The most common symptoms are pain in the back and the sides (between the ribs and hips), and headaches. The dull pain can be temporary or persistent, mild or severe.

People with autosomal dominant PKD also can experience the following:

- Urinary tract infections

- Hematuria (blood in the urine)

- Liver and pancreatic cysts

- Abnormal heart valves

- High blood pressure

- Kidney stones

- Aneurysms (bulges in the walls of blood vessels) in the brain

- Diverticulosis (small sacs on the colon)

How Is Autosomal Dominant PKD Diagnosed?

To diagnose autosomal dominant PKD, a doctor typically observes three or more kidney cysts using ultrasound imaging. The diagnosis is strengthened by a family history of autosomal dominant PKD and the presence of cysts in other organs. An ultrasound imaging device passes harmless sound waves through the body to detect possible kidney cysts.

In most cases of autosomal dominant PKD, the person's physical condition appears normal for many years, even decades, so the disease can go unnoticed. Physical checkups and blood and urine tests may not lead to diagnosis. The slow, undetected progression is why some people live for many years without knowing they have autosomal dominant PKD.

Once cysts have formed, however, diagnosis is possible with imaging technology. Ultrasound, which passes sound waves through the body to create a picture of the kidneys, is used most often. Ultrasound imaging employs no injected dyes or radiation and is safe for all patients including pregnant women. It can also detect cysts in the kidneys of a fetus.

More powerful and expensive imaging methods such as computed tomography (CT scan) and magnetic resonance imaging (MRI) also can detect cysts, but these methods usually are not required because ultrasound provides adequate information. CT scans require x rays and sometimes injected dyes.

In the future, DNA testing will be able to confirm a diagnosis of autosomal dominant PKD before cysts develop.

How Is Autosomal Dominant PKD Treated?

Although a cure for autosomal dominant PKD is not available, treatment can ease the symptoms and prolong life.

Pain

A doctor will first suggest over-the-counter pain medications, such as aspirin or Tylenol. For most but not all cases of severe pain, surgery to shrink cysts can relieve pain in the back and flanks. However, surgery provides only temporary relief and does not slow the disease's progression, in many cases, toward kidney failure.

Headaches that are severe or that seem to feel different from other headaches might be caused by aneurysms, or swollen blood vessels, in the brain. Headaches also can be caused by high blood pressure. People with autosomal dominant PKD should see a doctor if they have severe or recurring headaches--even before considering over-the-counter pain medications.

Urinary Tract Infections

Patients with autosomal dominant PKD tend to have frequent urinary tract infections, which can be treated with antibiotics. People with the disease should seek treatment for urinary tract infections immediately, because infection can spread from the urinary tract to the cysts in the kidneys. Cyst infections are difficult to treat because many antibiotics do not penetrate into the cysts. However, some antibiotics are effective.

High Blood Pressure

Keeping blood pressure under control can slow the effects of autosomal dominant PKD. Lifestyle changes and various medications can lower high blood pressure. Patients should ask their doctors about such treatments. Sometimes proper diet and exercise are enough to keep blood pressure low.

End-Stage Renal Disease

Because kidneys are essential for life, people with ESRD must seek one of two options for replacing kidney functions: dialysis or transplantation. In hemodialysis, blood is circulated into an external machine, where it is cleaned before reentering the body; in peritoneal dialysis, a fluid is introduced into the abdomen, where it absorbs wastes, and it is then removed. Transplantation of healthy kidneys into ESRD patients has become a common and successful procedure. Healthy (non-PKD) kidneys transplanted into PKD patients do not develop cysts.

What Is Autosomal Recessive PKD?

Autosomal recessive PKD is caused by a particular genetic flaw that is different from the genetic flaw that causes autosomal dominant PKD. Parents who do not have the disease can have a child with the disease if both parents carry the abnormal gene and both pass the gene to their baby. The chance of this happening (when both parents carry the abnormal gene) is one in four. If only one parent carries the abnormal gene, the baby cannot get the disease.

The symptoms of autosomal recessive PKD can begin before birth, so it is often called "infantile PKD." Children born with autosomal recessive PKD usually develop kidney failure within a few years. Severity of the disease varies. Babies with the worst cases die hours or days after birth. Children with an infantile version may have sufficient renal function for normal activities for a few years. People with the juvenile version may live into their teens and twenties and usually will have liver problems as well.

What Are the Symptoms of Autosomal Recessive PKD?

Children with autosomal recessive PKD experience high blood pressure, urinary tract infections, and frequent urination. The disease usually affects the liver, spleen, and pancreas, resulting in low blood-cell counts, varicose veins, and hemorrhoids. Because kidney function is crucial for early physical development, children with autosomal recessive PKD are usually smaller than average size.

How Is Autosomal Recessive PKD Diagnosed?

Ultrasound imaging of the fetus or newborn baby reveals cysts in the kidneys but does not distinguish between the cysts of autosomal recessive and autosomal dominant PKD. Ultrasound examination of kidneys of relatives can be helpful; for example, a parent or grandparent with autosomal dominant PKD cysts could help confirm diagnosis of autosomal dominant PKD in a fetus or child. (It is extremely rare, although not impossible, for a person with autosomal recessive PKD to become a parent.) Because autosomal recessive PKD tends to scar the liver, ultrasound imaging of the liver also aids in diagnosis.

How Is Autosomal Recessive PKD Treated?

Medicines can control high blood pressure in autosomal recessive PKD, and antibiotics can control urinary tract infections. Eating increased amounts of nutritious food improves growth in children with autosomal recessive PKD. In some cases, growth hormones are used. In response to kidney failure, autosomal recessive PKD patients must receive dialysis or transplantation.

Genetic Diseases

Genes are segments of DNA, the long molecules that reside in the nuclei of your body's cells. The genes, through complex processes, cause chemical activities that lead to growth and maintenance of the body. At conception, DNA (and therefore genes) from both parents are passed to the child.

A genetic disease occurs when one or both parents pass abnormal genes to a child at conception. If receiving an abnormal gene from just one parent is enough to produce a disease in the child, the disease is said to have dominant inheritance. If receiving abnormal genes from both parents is needed to produce disease in the child, the disease is said to be recessive.

The chance of acquiring a dominant disease (one gene copy is enough) is higher than the chance of acquiring a recessive disease (two gene copies are needed). A child who receives only one gene copy for a recessive disease at conception will not develop the genetic disease (such as autosomal recessive PKD), but could pass the gene to the following generation.

What Is Acquired Cystic Kidney Disease

ACKD develops in kidneys with long-term damage and bad scarring, so it often is associated with dialysis and end-stage renal disease. About 90 percent of people on dialysis for 5 years develop ACKD. People with ACKD can have any underlying kidney disease, such as glomerulonephritis or kidney disease of diabetes.

The cysts of ACKD may bleed. Kidney tumors, including kidney (renal) cancer, can develop in people with ACKD. Renal cancer is rare yet occurs at least twice as often in ACKD patients as in the general population.

How Is ACKD Diagnosed?

Patients with ACKD usually seek help because they notice blood in their urine (hematuria). The cysts bleed into the urinary system, which discolors urine. Diagnosis is confirmed using ultrasound, CT scan, or MRI of the kidneys.

How Is ACKD Treated?

Most ACKD patients are already receiving treatment for kidney problems. In rare cases, surgery is used to stop bleeding of cysts and to remove tumors or suspected tumors.

The Search for PKD Genes

Scientists have not determined the processes that trigger formation of PKD cysts. However, in recent years progress has been made in understanding the abnormal genes responsible for autosomal dominant and autosomal recessive PKD. Scientists have not yet developed clinical tests that determine whether a person carries a PKD gene.

In 1985, scientists narrowed their hunt for a PKD gene to a particular portion of human chromosome 16. In 1994, they precisely identified a gene associated with the vast majority of cases of autosomal dominant PKD. They named the gene "PKD1," knowing that one or more additional genes for autosomal dominant PKD have yet to be found. By 1995, scientists had produced a map of the PKD1 gene, showing all of its molecular components.

Scientists have continued to search for the autosomal recessive PKD gene. By 1995, they knew that a gene responsible for at least some cases of autosomal recessive PKD resides on chromosome 6.

Scientists will study PKD genes to learn their effects on chemical processes in the body. Knowing the effects will lead to better treatments for the diseases. Eventually, scientists may be able to correct genetic defects, eliminating the diseases entirely.

Points to Remember

The three types of PKD are:

- A common, inherited form that usually causes symptoms in midlife.
- A rare, inherited form that usually causes symptoms in early childhood.
- A noninherited form associated with long-term kidney problems, dialysis, and old age.

The signs of PKD include:

- Pain in the back and lower sides
- Headaches
- Urinary tract infections
- Blood in the urine
- Cysts in the kidneys and other organs

Diagnosis of PKD is obtained by:

- Ultrasound imaging of kidney cysts
- Ultrasound imaging of cysts in other organs
- Family medical history

PKD has no cure. Treatments include:

- Medicine and surgery to reduce pain
- Antibiotics to resolve infections
- Dialysis and transplantation to replace functions of failed kidneys

Additional Resources

For more information, contact:

Polycystic Kidney Disease Foundation
4901 Main Street
Suite 200
Kansas City, MO 64112
1-800-753-2873

American Association of Kidney Patients
100 South Ashley Drive
Suite 280
Tampa, FL 33602
1-800-749-2257

National Kidney Foundation
30 East 33rd Street
New York, NY 10016
1-800-622-9010

National Kidney and Urologic Diseases Information Clearinghouse
3 Information Way
Bethesda, MD 20892-3580
Email: nkudic@info.niddk.nih.gov
The National Kidney and Urologic Diseases Information Clearinghouse (NKUDIC) is a service of the National Institute of Diabetes and Digestive and Kidney Diseases (NIDDK). The NIDDK is part of the National Institutes of Health under the U.S. Department of Health and Human Services. Established in 1987, the clearinghouse provides information about diseases of the kidneys and urologic system to people with kidney and urologic disorders and to their families, health care professionals, and the public. NKUDIC answers inquiries, develops and distributes publications, and works closely with professional and patient organizations and Government agencies to coordinate resources about kidney and urologic diseases. Publications produced by the clearinghouse are carefully reviewed by both NIDDK scientists and outside experts.

More Guideline Sources

The guideline above on polycystic kidney disease is only one example of the kind of material that you can find online and free of charge. The remainder of this chapter will direct you to other sources which either publish or can help you find additional guidelines on topics related to polycystic kidney disease. Many of the guidelines listed below address topics that may be of particular relevance to your specific situation or of special interest to only some patients with polycystic kidney disease. Due to space limitations these sources are listed in a concise manner. Do not hesitate to consult the following sources by either using the Internet hyperlink provided, or, in cases where the contact information is provided, contacting the publisher or author directly.

Topic Pages: MEDLINEplus

For patients wishing to go beyond guidelines published by specific Institutes of the NIH, the National Library of Medicine has created a vast and patient-oriented healthcare information portal called MEDLINEplus. Within this Internet-based system are "health topic pages." You can think of a health topic page as a guide to patient guides. To access this system, log on to **http://www.nlm.nih.gov/medlineplus/healthtopics.html**.

If you do not find topics of interest when browsing health topic pages, then you can choose to use the advanced search utility of MEDLINEplus at **http://www.nlm.nih.gov/medlineplus/advancedsearch.html**. This utility is similar to the NIH Search Utility, with the exception that it only includes material linked within the MEDLINEplus system (mostly patient-oriented information). It also has the disadvantage of generating unstructured results. We recommend, therefore, that you use this method only if you have a very targeted search.

The Combined Health Information Database (CHID)

CHID Online is a reference tool that maintains a database directory of thousands of journal articles and patient education guidelines on polycystic kidney disease and related conditions. One of the advantages of CHID over other sources is that it offers summaries that describe the guidelines available, including contact information and pricing. CHID's general Web site is **http://chid.nih.gov/**. To search this database, go to **http://chid.nih.gov/detail/detail.html**. In particular, you can use the advanced search options to look up pamphlets, reports, brochures, and information kits. The following was recently posted in this archive:

- **Polycystic Kidney Disease: The Most Common Life-Threatening Genetic Disease**

  Source: Kansas City, MO: Polycystic Kidney Research Foundation. 200x. [7 p.].

  Contact: Available from KD Foundation. 4901 Main Street, Suite 200, Kansas City, MO 64112-2634. (800) 753-2873 or (816) 931-2600. Fax: (816) 931-8655. E-mail: pkdcure@pkrfoundation.org. Website: www.kumc.edu/pkrf/. Price: Single copy free.

  Summary: Polycystic kidney disease (PKD) is a disease that comes in two hereditary forms: autosomal dominant (ADPKD), the most common of all life threatening genetic diseases, or autosomal recessive (ARPKD), a relatively rare disease that often causes significant mortality in the first month of life. This brochure describes PKD and the work of the PKD Foundation, formerly called the Polycystic Kidney Research Foundation, an organization devoted to improving clinical treatment and discovering a cure for PKD. With the presence of PKD, cysts develop in both kidneys. There may be just a few cysts or many, and the cysts may range in size from a pinhead to the size of a grapefruit. Cysts are sacs of fluid that cause the kidney to enlarge and can hinder its filtering ability. Cysts also squeeze on blood vessels, forcing the pressure to rise. Beyond high blood pressure, symptoms of PKD include fatigue, frequent urination, blood in the urine, headaches, kidney stones, or urinary tract infections. ADPKD is not limited to the kidneys; common complications can include abnormalities in the vascular and cardiac systems. There are three main clinical tests used to diagnose PKD: ultrasound, computed tomography (CT), or magnetic resonance imaging (MRI). Current research demonstrates that a person with ADPKD may play a major role in controlling the disease with regular health care maintenance, a good diet, and regular exercise. The booklet describes many of the PKD Foundation's activities in research funding and advances, public awareness, and education. The booklet concludes with an invitation for readers to join the PKD Foundation and send a donation to support the work of this organization. 2 figures.

- **Your Child, Your Family and Autosomal Recessive Polycystic Kidney Disease. 2nd ed**

  Source: Kansas City, MO: Polycystic Kidney Research Foundation. 1996. 26 p.

Contact: Available from Polycystic Kidney Research Foundation. 4901 Main Street, Suite 320, Kansas City, MO 64112-2674. (800) PKD-CURE or (816) 931-2600. Fax (816) 931-8655. World Wide Web: http://www.kumc.edu/pkrf/. Price: $10.00 (members); $15.00 (for nonmembers).

Summary: This detailed booklet is designed to educate families about autosomal recessive polycystic kidney disease (ARPKD), which is sometimes referred to as infantile polycystic kidney disease. The booklet explains how the kidneys work; how ARPKD affects the kidneys and the liver; the genetics of ARPKD, which occurs in 1 to 2 of every 10,000 births; diagnosis and prenatal genetic testing; and the differences between ARPKD and other kinds of kidney disease. The authors discuss the major health problems in ARPKD, treatment, outlook, how to ensure appropriate medical care, family issues, and current research. 7 figures.

- **Polycystic Kidney Disease**

Source: New York, NY: National Kidney Foundation, Inc. 1990. 2p.

Contact: National Kidney Foundation, Inc. 30 East 33rd Street, New York, NY 10016. (800) 622-9010. Price: Single Copy free. Order No. 08-45.

Summary: This brochure briefly describes Polycystic Kidney Disease (PKD), including its symptoms; diagnosis, via computer tomography (CAT scan), ultrasonography, and blood testing; management of the disease through control of high blood pressure; and the effects of PKD on kidney function. The brochure provides a brief discussion of diet, exercise, and pregnancy and PKD, and highlights some research that is underway.

- **Autosomal Dominant Polycystic Kidney Disease (ADPKD)**

Source: Rochester, MN: Mayo Clinic. 1991. 10 p.

Contact: Available from Mayo Clinic. Patient and Health Education Center, 200 First Street, SW, Rochester, MN 55905. (507) 284-2511. Price: $2.75 plus shipping and handling. Order number MC 102/R391.

Summary: This booklet provides information to patients about autosomal dominant polycystic kidney disease (ADPKD). Written in a question and answer format, the booklet covers a definition of polycystic kidney disease; ADPKD as a genetic disease; how cysts develop in the kidneys; the symptoms of ADPKD; the spread of the cysts of ADPKD beyond the kidneys; the importance of screening family members for ADPKD; screening and diagnostic tests used; recommendations for people with

ADPKD; and research being done on this disease. The brochure concludes with a brief glossary.

The National Guideline Clearinghouse™

The National Guideline Clearinghouse™ offers hundreds of evidence-based clinical practice guidelines published in the United States and other countries. You can search their site located at **http://www.guideline.gov** by using the keyword "polycystic kidney disease" or synonyms. The following was recently posted:

- **Ultrasonographic examinations: indications and preparation of the patient.**

  Source: Finnish Medical Society Duodecim.; 2000 April 18; Various pagings

  http://www.guideline.gov/FRAMESETS/guideline_fs.asp?guideline=00 1844&sSearch_string=polycystic+kidney+disease

Healthfinder™

Healthfinder™ is an additional source sponsored by the U.S. Department of Health and Human Services which offers links to hundreds of other sites that contain healthcare information. This Web site is located at **http://www.healthfinder.gov**. Again, keyword searches can be used to find guidelines. The following was recently found in this database:

- **Polycystic Kidney Disease**

  Summary: Polycystic kidney disease (PKD) is a genetic disorder characterized by the growth of numerous cysts in the kidneys. The cysts are filled with fluid.

  Source: National Institute of Diabetes and Digestive and Kidney Diseases, National Institutes of Health

  http://www.healthfinder.gov/scripts/recordpass.asp?RecordType=0&R ecordID=6525

The NIH Search Utility

After browsing the references listed at the beginning of this chapter, you may want to explore the NIH Search Utility. This allows you to search for documents on over 100 selected Web sites that comprise the NIH-WEB-

SPACE. Each of these servers is "crawled" and indexed on an ongoing basis. Your search will produce a list of various documents, all of which will relate in some way to polycystic kidney disease. The drawbacks of this approach are that the information is not organized by theme and that the references are often a mix of information for professionals and patients. Nevertheless, a large number of the listed Web sites provide useful background information. We can only recommend this route, therefore, for relatively rare or specific disorders, or when using highly targeted searches. To use the NIH search utility, visit the following Web page: **http://search.nih.gov/index.html**.

Additional Web Sources

A number of Web sites that often link to government sites are available to the public. These can also point you in the direction of essential information. The following is a representative sample:

- AOL: **http://search.aol.com/cat.adp?id=168&layer=&from=subcats**

- drkoop.com®: **http://www.drkoop.com/conditions/ency/index.html**

- Family Village: **http://www.familyvillage.wisc.edu/specific.htm**

- Google: **http://directory.google.com/Top/Health/Conditions_and_Diseases/**

- Med Help International: **http://www.medhelp.org/HealthTopics/A.html**

- Open Directory Project: **http://dmoz.org/Health/Conditions_and_Diseases/**

- Yahoo.com: **http://dir.yahoo.com/Health/Diseases_and_Conditions/**

- WebMD®Health: **http://my.webmd.com/health_topics**

Vocabulary Builder

The material in this chapter may have contained a number of unfamiliar words. The following Vocabulary Builder introduces you to terms used in this chapter that have not been covered in the previous chapter:

Abdomen: That portion of the body that lies between the thorax and the pelvis. [NIH]

Aneurysm: A sac formed by the dilatation of the wall of an artery, a vein, or the heart. The chief signs of arterial aneurysm are the formation of a pulsating tumour, and often a bruit (aneurysmal bruit) heard over the swelling. Sometimes there are symptoms from pressure on contiguous parts. [EU]

Antibiotic: A chemical substance produced by a microorganism which has the capacity, in dilute solutions, to inhibit the growth of or to kill other microorganisms. Antibiotics that are sufficiently nontoxic to the host are used as chemotherapeutic agents in the treatment of infectious diseases of man, animals and plants. [EU]

Conception: The onset of pregnancy, marked by implantation of the blastocyst; the formation of a viable zygote. [EU]

Dyes: Chemical substances that are used to stain and color other materials. The coloring may or may not be permanent. Dyes can also be used as therapeutic agents and test reagents in medicine and scientific research. [NIH]

Endocrinology: A subspecialty of internal medicine concerned with the metabolism, physiology, and disorders of the endocrine system. [NIH]

Fatigue: The state of weariness following a period of exertion, mental or physical, characterized by a decreased capacity for work and reduced efficiency to respond to stimuli. [NIH]

Glomerulonephritis: A variety of nephritis characterized by inflammation of the capillary loops in the glomeruli of the kidney. It occurs in acute, subacute, and chronic forms and may be secondary to haemolytic streptococcal infection. Evidence also supports possible immune or autoimmune mechanisms. [EU]

Hematology: A subspecialty of internal medicine concerned with morphology, physiology, and pathology of the blood and blood-forming tissues. [NIH]

Hematuria: Presence of blood in the urine. [NIH]

Hemorrhoids: Varicosities of the hemorrhoidal venous plexuses. [NIH]

Hormones: Chemical substances having a specific regulatory effect on the activity of a certain organ or organs. The term was originally applied to substances secreted by various endocrine glands and transported in the bloodstream to the target organs. It is sometimes extended to include those substances that are not produced by the endocrine glands but that have similar effects. [NIH]

Hypertension: Persistently high arterial blood pressure. Various criteria for its threshold have been suggested, ranging from 140 mm. Hg systolic and 90 mm. Hg diastolic to as high as 200 mm. Hg systolic and 110 mm. Hg diastolic. Hypertension may have no known cause (essential or idiopathic h.) or be associated with other primary diseases (secondary h.). [EU]

Molecular: Of, pertaining to, or composed of molecules : a very small mass of matter. [EU]

Nephrons: The functional units of the kidney, consisting of the glomerulus and the attached tubule. [NIH]

Pancreas: A mixed exocrine and endocrine gland situated transversely across the posterior abdominal wall in the epigastric and hypochondriac regions. The endocrine portion is comprised of the islets of langerhans, while the exocrine portion is a compound acinar gland that secretes digestive enzymes. [NIH]

Prenatal: Existing or occurring before birth, with reference to the fetus. [EU]

Spectrum: A charted band of wavelengths of electromagnetic vibrations obtained by refraction and diffraction. By extension, a measurable range of activity, such as the range of bacteria affected by an antibiotic (antibacterial s.) or the complete range of manifestations of a disease. [EU]

Tomography: The recording of internal body images at a predetermined plane by means of the tomograph; called also body section roentgenography. [EU]

Toxicology: The science concerned with the detection, chemical composition, and pharmacologic action of toxic substances or poisons and the treatment and prevention of toxic manifestations. [NIH]

Transplantation: The grafting of tissues taken from the patient's own body or from another. [EU]

Ultrasonography: The visualization of deep structures of the body by recording the reflections of echoes of pulses of ultrasonic waves directed into the tissues. Use of ultrasound for imaging or diagnostic purposes employs frequencies ranging from 1.6 to 10 megahertz. [NIH]

Urology: A surgical specialty concerned with the study, diagnosis, and treatment of diseases of the urinary tract in both sexes and the genital tract in the male. It includes the specialty of andrology which addresses both male genital diseases and male infertility. [NIH]

Vascular: Pertaining to blood vessels or indicative of a copious blood supply. [EU]

Veins: The vessels carrying blood toward the heart. [NIH]

CHAPTER 2. SEEKING GUIDANCE

Overview

Some patients are comforted by the knowledge that a number of organizations dedicate their resources to helping people with polycystic kidney disease. These associations can become invaluable sources of information and advice. Many associations offer aftercare support, financial assistance, and other important services. Furthermore, healthcare research has shown that support groups often help people to better cope with their conditions.[8] In addition to support groups, your physician can be a valuable source of guidance and support. Therefore, finding a physician that can work with your unique situation is a very important aspect of your care.

In this chapter, we direct you to resources that can help you find patient organizations and medical specialists. We begin by describing how to find associations and peer groups that can help you better understand and cope with polycystic kidney disease. The chapter ends with a discussion on how to find a doctor that is right for you.

Associations and Polycystic Kidney Disease

As mentioned by the Agency for Healthcare Research and Quality, sometimes the emotional side of an illness can be as taxing as the physical side.[9] You may have fears or feel overwhelmed by your situation. Everyone has different ways of dealing with disease or physical injury. Your attitude, your expectations, and how well you cope with your condition can all

---

[8] Churches, synagogues, and other houses of worship might also have groups that can offer you the social support you need.
[9] This section has been adapted from **http://www.ahcpr.gov/consumer/diaginf5.htm**.

influence your well-being. This is true for both minor conditions and serious illnesses. For example, a study on female breast cancer survivors revealed that women who participated in support groups lived longer and experienced better quality of life when compared with women who did not participate. In the support group, women learned coping skills and had the opportunity to share their feelings with other women in the same situation.

In addition to associations or groups that your doctor might recommend, we suggest that you consider the following list (if there is a fee for an association, you may want to check with your insurance provider to find out if the cost will be covered):

- **Autosomal Recessive Polycystic Kidney Disease Family Support**

  Address: Autosomal Recessive Polycystic Kidney Disease Family Support 38 John Drive, Kirkwood, PA 17536-9523

  Telephone: (717) 529-6732 Toll-free: (800) 753-2873

  Fax: (717) 529-6732

  Email: None.

  Web Site: Non

  Background: Autosomal Recessive Polycystic Kidney Disease Family Support is a self-help organization dedicated to providing information and support to affected individuals and families, promoting professional and public awareness, and supporting research. Autosomal recessive polycystic kidney disease (ARPKD) is a rare inherited disorder that may be apparent at birth. Affected newborns often have poorly developed lungs, causing life-threatening complications in some cases. Infants with the disorder experience the development of multiple cysts in both kidneys, potentially causing severe enlargement of the kidneys. The progressive development of additional cysts and cyst enlargement may cause destruction of normal kidney tissue and associated kidney failure. Affected children may also experience abnormal widening of the liver's bile ducts, scarring around the ducts, and associated blockage of the liver's blood vessels (congenital hepatic fibrosis), which may cause enlargement of the liver and spleen, chronic bile duct infections, and eventual liver failure. In individuals with autosomal recessive polycystic kidney disease, the range and severity of associated symptoms and findings may vary greatly from case to case. Autosomal Recessive Polycystic Kidney Disease Family Support was established in 1993 and currently consists of approximately 100 members. The organization provides networking opportunities to affected families, conducts regular support group meetings with scheduled speakers, and offers a variety of educational materials including pamphlets and a regular newsletter. In addition, the organization is committed to promoting and supporting basic and clinical research and utilizing a database for research purposes.

Relevant area(s) of interest: Polycystic Kidney Disease

- **March of Dimes Birth Defects Foundation**

  Address: March of Dimes Birth Defects Foundation 1275 Mamaroneck Avenue, White Plains, NY 10605

  Telephone: (914) 428-7100 Toll-free: (888) 663-4637

  Fax: (914) 997-4763

  Email: resourcecenter@modimes.org

  Web Site: http://www.modimes.or

  Background: The March of Dimes Birth Defects Foundation is a national not-for- profit organization that was established in 1938. The mission of the Foundation is to improve the health of babies by preventing birth defects and infant mortality. Through the Campaign for Healthier Babies, the March of Dimes funds programs of research, community services, education, and advocacy. Educational programs that seek to prevent birth defects are important to the Foundation and to that end it produces a wide variety of printed informational materials and videos. The March of Dimes public health educational materials provide information encouraging health- enhancing behaviors that lead to a healthy pregnancy and a healthy baby.

  Relevant area(s) of interest: Medullary Cystic Disease, Polycystic Kidney Disease

- **PKR (Polycystic Kidney Research) Foundation**

  Address: PKR (Polycystic Kidney Research) Foundation 4901 Main St., Suite 200, Kansas City, MO 64112-2634

  Telephone: (816) 931-2600 Toll-free: (800) 753-2873

  Fax: (816) 931-8655

  Email: pkdcure@pkrfoundation.org

  Web Site: http://www.pkdcure.or

  Background: The PKR (Polycystic Kidney Research) Foundation is an international not-for-profit voluntary organization that was established in 1982. The Foundation is committed to providing emotional support and educational materials to people with Polycystic Kidney Disease and their families. The Foundation seeks to promote public awareness of polycystic kidney disease and raise funds that will support ongoing medical research into the causes, treatment, and prevention of this disease. The PKR Foundation conducts informational seminars and conferences; provides phone support for newly diagnosed affected individuals and publishes a quarterly newsletter. It assists in the formation and maintenance of new support groups and makes appropriate referrals to physicians who are familiar with this disorder.

Relevant area(s) of interest: Polycystic Kidney Disease

Finding More Associations

There are a number of directories that list additional medical associations that you may find useful. While not all of these directories will provide different information than what is listed above, by consulting all of them, you will have nearly exhausted all sources for patient associations.

The National Health Information Center (NHIC)

The National Health Information Center (NHIC) offers a free referral service to help people find organizations that provide information about polycystic kidney disease. For more information, see the NHIC's Web site at **http://www.health.gov/NHIC/** or contact an information specialist by calling 1-800-336-4797.

DIRLINE

A comprehensive source of information on associations is the DIRLINE database maintained by the National Library of Medicine. The database comprises some 10,000 records of organizations, research centers, and government institutes and associations which primarily focus on health and biomedicine. DIRLINE is available via the Internet at the following Web site: **http://dirline.nlm.nih.gov/**. Simply type in "polycystic kidney disease" (or a synonym) or the name of a topic, and the site will list information contained in the database on all relevant organizations.

The Combined Health Information Database

Another comprehensive source of information on healthcare associations is the Combined Health Information Database. Using the "Detailed Search" option, you will need to limit your search to "Organizations" and "polycystic kidney disease". Type the following hyperlink into your Web browser: **http://chid.nih.gov/detail/detail.html**. To find associations, use the drop boxes at the bottom of the search page where "You may refine your search by." For publication date, select "All Years." Then, select your preferred language and the format option "Organization Resource Sheet." By making these selections and typing in "polycystic kidney disease" (or synonyms) into the "For these words:" box, you will only receive results on organizations dealing with polycystic kidney disease. You should check back periodically with this database since it is updated every 3 months.

The National Organization for Rare Disorders, Inc.

The National Organization for Rare Disorders, Inc. has prepared a Web site that provides, at no charge, lists of associations organized by specific diseases. You can access this database at the following Web site: **http://www.rarediseases.org/cgi-bin/nord/searchpage**. Select the option called "Organizational Database (ODB)" and type "polycystic kidney disease" (or a synonym) in the search box.

Online Support Groups

In addition to support groups, commercial Internet service providers offer forums and chat rooms for people with different illnesses and conditions. WebMD®, for example, offers such a service at their Web site: **http://boards.webmd.com/roundtable**. These online self-help communities can help you connect with a network of people whose concerns are similar to yours. Online support groups are places where people can talk informally. If you read about a novel approach, consult with your doctor or other healthcare providers, as the treatments or discoveries you hear about may not be scientifically proven to be safe and effective.   The following Internet sites may be of particular ineterest:

- **Polycystic Kidney Disease Access Center**
  http://www.nhpress.com/pkd

- **Kansas Medical Center**
  http://www.kumc.edu/gec/support/

- **MedHelp**
  http://www.medhelp.org/HealthTopics/ Polycystic_Kidney_Disease.html

Finding Doctors

One of the most important aspects of your treatment will be the relationship between you and your doctor or specialist. All patients with polycystic kidney disease must go through the process of selecting a physician. While this process will vary from person to person, the Agency for Healthcare Research and Quality makes a number of suggestions, including the following:[10]

- If you are in a managed care plan, check the plan's list of doctors first.

- Ask doctors or other health professionals who work with doctors, such as hospital nurses, for referrals.

- Call a hospital's doctor referral service, but keep in mind that these services usually refer you to doctors on staff at that particular hospital. The services do not have information on the quality of care that these doctors provide.

- Some local medical societies offer lists of member doctors. Again, these lists do not have information on the quality of care that these doctors provide.

Additional steps you can take to locate doctors include the following:

- Check with the associations listed earlier in this chapter.

- Information on doctors in some states is available on the Internet at **http://www.docboard.org**. This Web site is run by "Administrators in Medicine," a group of state medical board directors.

- The American Board of Medical Specialties can tell you if your doctor is board certified. "Certified" means that the doctor has completed a training program in a specialty and has passed an exam, or "board," to assess his or her knowledge, skills, and experience to provide quality patient care in that specialty. Primary care doctors may also be certified as specialists. The AMBS Web site is located at **http://www.abms.org/newsearch.asp**.[11] You can also contact the ABMS by phone at 1-866-ASK-ABMS.

- You can call the American Medical Association (AMA) at 800-665-2882 for information on training, specialties, and board certification for many licensed doctors in the United States. This information also can be found

---

[10] This section is adapted from the AHRQ: **www.ahrq.gov/consumer/qntascii/qntdr.htm** .
[11] While board certification is a good measure of a doctor's knowledge, it is possible to receive quality care from doctors who are not board certified.

in "Physician Select" at the AMA's Web site: **http://www.ama-assn.org/aps/amahg.htm**.

Finding a Urologist

The American Urological Association (AUA) provides the public with a free-to-use "Find A Urologist" service to help patients find member urologists in their area. The database can be searched by physician name, city, U.S. State, or country and is available via the AUA's Web site located at **http://www.auanet.org/patient_info/find_urologist/index.cfm**. According to the AUA: "The American Urological Association is the professional association for urologists. As the premier professional association for the advancement of urologic patient care, the AUA is pleased to provide Find A Urologist, an on-line referral service for patients to use when looking for a urologist. All of our active members are certified by the American Board of Urology, which is an important distinction of the urologist's commitment to continuing education and superior patient care."[12]

If the previous sources did not meet your needs, you may want to log on to the Web site of the National Organization for Rare Disorders (NORD) at **http://www.rarediseases.org/**. NORD maintains a database of doctors with expertise in various rare diseases. The Metabolic Information Network (MIN), 800-945-2188, also maintains a database of physicians with expertise in various metabolic diseases.

Selecting Your Doctor[13]

When you have compiled a list of prospective doctors, call each of their offices. First, ask if the doctor accepts your health insurance plan and if he or she is taking new patients. If the doctor is not covered by your plan, ask yourself if you are prepared to pay the extra costs. The next step is to schedule a visit with your chosen physician. During the first visit you will have the opportunity to evaluate your doctor and to find out if you feel comfortable with him or her. Ask yourself, did the doctor:

- Give me a chance to ask questions about polycystic kidney disease?
- Really listen to my questions?

[12] Quotation taken from the AACE's Web site: **http://www.aace.com/memsearch.php**.
[13] This section has been adapted from the AHRQ: **www.ahrq.gov/consumer/qntascii/qntdr.htm**.

- Answer in terms I understood?

- Show respect for me?

- Ask me questions?

- Make me feel comfortable?

- Address the health problem(s) I came with?

- Ask me my preferences about different kinds of treatments for polycystic kidney disease?

- Spend enough time with me?

Trust your instincts when deciding if the doctor is right for you. But remember, it might take time for the relationship to develop. It takes more than one visit for you and your doctor to get to know each other.

Working with Your Doctor[4]

Research has shown that patients who have good relationships with their doctors tend to be more satisfied with their care and have better results. Here are some tips to help you and your doctor become partners:

- You know important things about your symptoms and your health history. Tell your doctor what you think he or she needs to know.

- It is important to tell your doctor personal information, even if it makes you feel embarrassed or uncomfortable.

- Bring a "health history" list with you (and keep it up to date).

- Always bring any medications you are currently taking with you to the appointment, or you can bring a list of your medications including dosage and frequency information. Talk about any allergies or reactions you have had to your medications.

- Tell your doctor about any natural or alternative medicines you are taking.

- Bring other medical information, such as x-ray films, test results, and medical records.

- Ask questions. If you don't, your doctor will assume that you understood everything that was said.

---

[4] This section has been adapted from the AHRQ: **www.ahrq.gov/consumer/qntascii/qntdr.htm**.

- Write down your questions before your visit. List the most important ones first to make sure that they are addressed.

- Consider bringing a friend with you to the appointment to help you ask questions. This person can also help you understand and/or remember the answers.

- Ask your doctor to draw pictures if you think that this would help you understand.

- Take notes. Some doctors do not mind if you bring a tape recorder to help you remember things, but always ask first.

- Let your doctor know if you need more time. If there is not time that day, perhaps you can speak to a nurse or physician assistant on staff or schedule a telephone appointment.

- Take information home. Ask for written instructions. Your doctor may also have brochures and audio and videotapes that can help you.

- After leaving the doctor's office, take responsibility for your care. If you have questions, call. If your symptoms get worse or if you have problems with your medication, call. If you had tests and do not hear from your doctor, call for your test results. If your doctor recommended that you have certain tests, schedule an appointment to get them done. If your doctor said you should see an additional specialist, make an appointment.

By following these steps, you will enhance the relationship you will have with your physician.

Broader Health-Related Resources

In addition to the references above, the NIH has set up guidance Web sites that can help patients find healthcare professionals. These include:[15]

- Caregivers:
  http://www.nlm.nih.gov/medlineplus/caregivers.html

- Choosing a Doctor or Healthcare Service:
  http://www.nlm.nih.gov/medlineplus/choosingadoctororhealthcareserv ice.html

---

[15] You can access this information at:
http://www.nlm.nih.gov/medlineplus/healthsystem.html.

- Hospitals and Health Facilities:
  http://www.nlm.nih.gov/medlineplus/healthfacilities.html

Vocabulary Builder

The following vocabulary builder provides definitions of words used in this chapter that have not been defined in previous chapters:

Bile: An emulsifying agent produced in the liver and secreted into the duodenum. Its composition includes bile acids and salts, cholesterol, and electrolytes. It aids digestion of fats in the duodenum. [NIH]

Fibrosis: The formation of fibrous tissue; fibroid or fibrous degeneration [EU]

Medullary: Pertaining to the marrow or to any medulla; resembling marrow. [EU]

Progressive: Advancing; going forward; going from bad to worse; increasing in scope or severity. [EU]

PART II: ADDITIONAL RESOURCES AND ADVANCED MATERIAL

ABOUT PART II

In Part II, we introduce you to additional resources and advanced research on polycystic kidney disease. All too often, patients who conduct their own research are overwhelmed by the difficulty in finding and organizing information. The purpose of the following chapters is to provide you an organized and structured format to help you find additional information resources on polycystic kidney disease. In Part II, as in Part I, our objective is not to interpret the latest advances on polycystic kidney disease or render an opinion. Rather, our goal is to give you access to original research and to increase your awareness of sources you may not have already considered. In this way, you will come across the advanced materials often referred to in pamphlets, books, or other general works. Once again, some of this material is technical in nature, so consultation with a professional familiar with polycystic kidney disease is suggested.

CHAPTER 3. STUDIES ON POLYCYSTIC KIDNEY DISEASE

Overview

Every year, academic studies are published on polycystic kidney disease or related conditions. Broadly speaking, there are two types of studies. The first are peer reviewed. Generally, the content of these studies has been reviewed by scientists or physicians. Peer-reviewed studies are typically published in scientific journals and are usually available at medical libraries. The second type of studies is non-peer reviewed. These works include summary articles that do not use or report scientific results. These often appear in the popular press, newsletters, or similar periodicals.

In this chapter, we will show you how to locate peer-reviewed references and studies on polycystic kidney disease. We will begin by discussing research that has been summarized and is free to view by the public via the Internet. We then show you how to generate a bibliography on polycystic kidney disease and teach you how to keep current on new studies as they are published or undertaken by the scientific community.

The Combined Health Information Database

The Combined Health Information Database summarizes studies across numerous federal agencies. To limit your investigation to research studies and polycystic kidney disease, you will need to use the advanced search options. First, go to **http://chid.nih.gov/index.html**. From there, select the "Detailed Search" option (or go directly to that page with the following hyperlink: **http://chid.nih.gov/detail/detail.html**). The trick in extracting studies is found in the drop boxes at the bottom of the search page where "You may refine your search by." Select the dates and language you prefer, and the format option "Journal Article." At the top of the search form, select the number of records you would like to see (we recommend 100) and check the box to display "whole records." We recommend that you type in "polycystic kidney disease" (or synonyms) into the "For these words:" box. Consider using the option "anywhere in record" to make your search as broad as possible. If you want to limit the search to only a particular field, such as the title of the journal, then select this option in the "Search in these fields" drop box. The following is a sample of what you can expect from this type of search:

- **Inherited Renal and Genitourinary Disorders: Autosomal Recessive Polycystic Kidney Disease**

  Source: Journal of Rare Diseases. 3(6): 23-25. November-December 1997.

  Contact: Available from Dowden Publishing Company. 110 Summit Avenue, Montvale, NJ 07645. (800) 707-7040 or (201) 391-9100. Fax (201) 391-2778.

  Summary: This article reviews autosomal recessive polycystic kidney disease (ARPKD), one of the most frequently observed hereditary renal cystic disorders in children. The author summarizes recent research on this disease. Genetic studies have recently designated the only known locus for this condition to a specific chromosome (6p21-p12). A recent review (Popovic-Rolovic et al, 1996) covers new information on genetics and cellular malformations responsible for the growth and development of kidney cysts; these authors highlight the identification of the location of the gene for autosomal dominant PKD (ADPKD) 1 and 2 on the short arms of chromosome 16 and 4, respectively. Zerres and others present a prospective nonrandom study of 115 children (66 male, 49 female) with ARPKD who were followed for an average of nearly 5 years. Most of the children survived the neonatal period; drug therapy for hypertension was necessary in 70 percent of cases; reduced glomerular filtration rates (GFR, a measure of kidney function) were seen in 72 percent of patients; 11 children progressed to end stage renal disease (ESRD). The authors note that long term prognosis in pediatric cases of ARPKD is more encouraging than generally stated in the literature. The author of this summary notes advances in fetal diagnosis of ARPKD, including the standard use of ultrasonography and the indications for further testing. 6 references.

- **Polycystic Kidney Disease (PKD)**

  Source: American Family Physician. 53(3): 935-936. February 15, 1996.

Summary: This patient education handout provides information on polycystic kidney disease (PKD), an inherited disease in which cysts grow in the kidneys. Written in a question and answer format, the handout covers how PKD can affect one's daily life, PKD-related hypertension (high blood pressure), PKD and kidney failure, other organs that can be hurt by PKD, the symptoms of the disease, diagnostic considerations, PKD in infants, genetic considerations, diagnostic tests, and treatment options. The handout concludes with the names, addresses, and telephone numbers of two resource organizations: Polycystic Kidney Research Foundation and the National Kidney Foundation.

- **Analysis of the Genomic Sequence for the Autosomal Dominant Polycystic Kidney Disease (PKD1) Gene Predicts the Presence of a Leucine-Rich Repeat**

Source: Human Molecular Genetics. 4(4): 575-582. April 1995.

Contact: Available from IRL Press. Oxford University Press, Inc. 2001 Evans Road, Cary, NC 27513.

Summary: This article reports on research in which the complete genomic sequence of the gene responsible for the predominant form of polycystic kidney disease (PKD1) was determined, in order to provide a framework for understanding the biology and evolution of the gene, and to aid in the development of molecular diagnostics. The authors describe how the DNA sequence of a 54 kb interval immediately upstream of the poly(A) addition signal sequence of the PKD1 transcript was determined and analyzed using computer methods. A leucine-rich repeat (LRR) motif was identified within the resulting predicted protein sequence of the PKD gene. By analogy with other LRR-containing proteins, this may explain some of the disease-related renal alterations such as mislocalization of membrane protein constituents and changes in the extracellular matrix organization. 4 figures. 71 references. (AA-M).

- **Genetics and Physiology of Polycystic Kidney Disease**

Source: Seminars in Nephrology. 21(2): 107-123. March 2001.

Contact: Available from W.B. Saunders Company. Periodicals Department, 6277 Sea Harbor Drive, Orlando, FL 32887-4800. (800) 654-2452.

Summary: Autosomal dominant polycystic kidney disease (ADPKD) is a major, inherited disorder that is characterized by the growth of large, fluid filled cysts from the tubules and collecting ducts of affected kidneys, and by a number of extrarenal manifestations including liver and pancreatic cysts, hypertension, heart valve defects, and cerebral (brain) and aortic aneurysms. This article explores the genetics and physiology of polycystic kidney disease. Mutations in either of 2 different genes (PKD1 or PKD2) give rise to ADPKD. The authors note that most mutations identified in affected families appear to inactivate the PKD genes, and they discuss accumulating evidence that suggests that a 2 hit mechanism, in which the normal PKD1 or PKD2 allele is also mutated, may be required for cyst growth. The pathogenesis of cyst formation is currently thought to involve increased cell proliferation, fluid accumulation, and basement membrane remodeling. In contrast to normal kidney cells whose cell proliferation is inhibited by cyclic AMP (adenosine monophosphate), ADPKD cells are stimulated to proliferate. Cyclic AMP and growth factors, including epidermal growth factor, have complementary effects to accelerate the enlargement of ADPKD cysts, and thereby to contribute to the progression of the disease. The authors hope that this knowledge will facilitate the discovery of inhibitors of signal transduction cascades that can be used in the treatment of ADPKD. 3 figures. 234 references.

- **Molecular Genetics and Pathogenesis of Autosomal Dominant Polycystic Kidney Disease**

Source: in Coggins, C.H.; Hancock, E.W., Eds. Annual Review of Medicine: Selected Topics in the Clinical Sciences, Volume 52. Palo Alto, CA: Annual Reviews Inc. 2001. p. 93-123.

Contact: Available from Annual Reviews Inc. 4139 El Camino Way, P.O. Box 10139, Palo Alto, CA 94303-0139. (800) 523-8635. Fax: (415) 855-9815. Price: $47. ISBN: 0824305450.

Summary: Autosomal dominant polycystic kidney disease (ADPKD) is a common and systemic disease characterized by formation of focal cysts in the kidneys. Rapid progress has been made over the past few years in identifying the genes responsible for the vast majority of cases of ADPKD, in unraveling the underlying mutations, in localizing the gene products at the cellular and subcellular levels, and in developing animal models that reproduce many of the disease features. This article considers the molecular genetics and pathogenesis of ADPKD. Of the three potential causes of cysts, downstream obstruction, compositional changes in extracellular matrix, and proliferation of partially dedifferentiated cells, evidence strongly supports the latter as the primary abnormality. In the vast majority of cases, the disease is caused by mutations in PKD1 or PKD2, and appears to be recessive at the cellular level. Somatic second hits in the normal allele of cells containing the germ line mutation initiate or accelerate formation of cysts. PKD1 and

PKD2 encode a putative adhesive ion channel regulatory protein and an ion channel respectively. The two proteins interact directly in vitro. Their cellular and subcellular localization suggest that they may also function independently in a common signaling pathway that may involve the membrane skeleton and that links cell to cell and cell to matrix adhesion to the development of cell polarity. 2 figures. 225 references.

- **Nephrolithiasis Associated with Autosomal Dominant Polycystic Kidney Disease: Contemporary Urological Management**

  Source: Journal of Urology. 163(3): 726-729. March 2000.

  Contact: Available from Lippincott Williams and Wilkins. 12107 Insurance Way, Hagerstown, MD 21740. (800) 638-3030 or (301) 714-2334. Fax (301) 824-7290.

  Summary: This article reports on a study undertaken to evaluate the role of contemporary urological intervention in patients with nephrolithiasis (kidney stones) associated with autosomal dominant polycystic kidney disease (ADPKD). Intervention for upper tract stones associated with autosomal dominant polycystic kidney disease was performed in 5 women and 2 men, aged 29 to 65 years old (mean age 47 years). Indications for intervention consisted of flank pain in 6 patients or hematuria (blood in the urine) in 2 patients. A total of 12 procedures (mean 1.7 per patient) were performed, including shock wave lithotripsy (ESWL) in 6 patients, percutaneous nephrolithotomy (surgery 'through the skin' to remove the stones) in 2 patients, retrograde endoscopy or manipulation in 3 patients, and extended pyelonephrolithotomy in 1 patient. All patients were rendered stone free or had only residual 'dust.' Hospital stay for 5 patients was 1 night or less, and there were no complications. Renal (kidney) function for each patient was stable or improved as measured by serum creatinine. The authors conclude that most patients with ADPKD who require intervention for kidney stones can be safely and effectively treated with essentially any or all contemporary, minimally invasive techniques. The choice of intervention can be based primarily on size and location of the upper tract stones rather than the associated presence of polycystic kidneys. 3 figures. 1 table. 7 references.

- **Pathogenesis of Autosomal Dominant Polycystic Kidney Disease: An Update**

  Source: Current Opinion in Nephrology and Hypertension. 9(4): 385-394. July 2000.

Contact: Available from Lippincott Williams and Wilkins. P.O. Box 1600, Hagerstown, MD 21741. (800) 638-3030 or (301) 223-2300. Fax (301) 223-2400. Website: www.currentopinion.com.

Summary: The identification of PKD1 and PKD2, the two major genes responsible for autosomal dominant polycystic kidney disease (ADPKD), are the important discoveries upon which much of the current investigation into the pathogenesis of this common heritable disease is based. This article updates readers on the pathogenesis of ADPKD. A major mechanistic insight was achieved with the discovery that ADPKD occurs by a two hit mechanism requiring somatic inactivation of the normal allele in individual polarized epithelial cells. Most recent advances are focused on the function of the respective protein products (polycystin 1 and polycystin 2). Indirect evidence supports and interaction between polycystin 1 and 2, but the authors note that it is unlikely that they work in concert in all tissues and at all times. The authors review the similarities and differences of these protein products and their role in understanding ADPKD. The authors describe ongoing research projects and note that the understanding of this disease is reaching a critical stage at which rational treatment approaches may become reality. Identification of targets for conditional lethality in cyst lining cells will be a major step in modifying the course of this disease. 2 figures. 69 references.

- **Autosomal Dominant Polycystic Kidney Disease: Pathophysiology and Treatment**

Source: ANNA Journal. American Nephrology Nurses Association Journal. 24(1): 45-51. February 1997.

Contact: Available from American Nephrology Nurses' Association. East Holly Avenue, Box 56, Pitman, NJ 08071-0056. (609) 256-2320.

Summary: Once viewed as a hopelessly incurable disease, autosomal dominant polycystic kidney disease (ADPKD) has been given a great deal of attention as geneticists search for ADPKD genes, and cell biologists are studying and understanding cyst formation. This continuing education nursing article covers the pathophysiology and treatment of ADPKD. Alterations in cellular growth, secretion, and extracellular matrix all participate in cystogenesis. The disease is a systemic disorder that may affect multiple organ systems. Manifestations of ADPKD in renal and extrarenal systems may be challenging problems in the management of these patients. Renal manifestations include renal cysts, decreased renal concentrating ability, increased renin production, increased erythropoietin production, hypertension, hematuria, acute and chronic pain, urinary tract infection, and nephrolithiasis. Extrarenal manifestations include hepatic cysts, pancreatic cysts, cardiac valvular abnormalities, intracranial aneurysm, thoracic aortic aneurysm, abdominal aortic aneurysm, ovarian cysts, pineal cysts, splenic cysts, and testicular cysts. The authors describe the medical treatment for these manifestations of ADPKD. The authors also consider the recommended nursing interventions for patients with ADPKD and their families. Readers can qualify for 2.0 continuing education credits by completing and passing the posttest. 2 figures. 1 table. 27 references. (AA-M).

- **Autosomal Dominant Polycystic Kidney Disease: A Genetic Perspective**

Source: Nephrology. 3(5): 387-395. October 1997.

Contact: Available from Blackwell Science. Commerce Place, 350 Main Street, Malden, MA 02148-5018. (617) 388-8273.

Summary: This article reviews recent important advances in understanding autosomal dominant polycystic kidney disease (ADPKD), a common genetic disease. The major ADPKD genes, PKD1 and PKD2, have been identified and characterized in the past 3 years. The predicted PKD1 protein, called polycystin, has a large extracellular region containing motifs involved in protein-protein and protein-carbohydrate interactions. The PKD1 protein is attached to the membrane with multiple transmembrane regions. PKD2 is a small integral membrane protein with cytoplasmic N and C termini, 6 transmembrane domains, and a region of homology with polycystin. The similarity of PKD2 to voltage-gated ion channels and an area of homology between polycystin and a receptor for egg jelly protein, which is thought to regulate ion channels, suggests a role for the ADPKD proteins in ion transport. The PKD1 and PKD2 genes are expressed in most tissues, and polycystin has been localized to tubular epithelial structures in the fetal and adult kidney. A specific syndrome due to a deletion of PKD1 and the adjacent TSC2 gene is associated with early onset polycystic kidney disease and tuberous sclerosis. 2 figures. 99 references. (AA-M).

- **Polycystic Kidney Disease 1 (PKD-1) Gene: An Important Clue In the Study of Renal Cyst Formation**

Source: Journal of the Royal College of Physicians of London. 31(2): 141-146. March-April 1997.

Contact: Available from Royal College of Physicians. Publications Department, 11 Saint Andrews Place, Regent's Park, London NW1 4LE. 0171 935 1174. Fax 0171 487 5218.

Summary: A major breakthrough in the study of polycystic kidney diseases came in 1985 when polycystic kidney disease 1 (PKD1), the major gene responsible in almost 90 percent of patients with autosomal dominant polycystic kidney disease (ADPKD) was linked to the short arm of chromosome 16 (16p). This article reviews the present state of knowledge of PKD1, addressing three areas of interest: the function of polycystin (the protein encoded by PKD1), the reasons for the marked phenotypic variability seen in individuals with PKD1, and the molecular basis of cyst formation in PKD1. The author first discusses the problems that continue to face researchers in this field. The author notes that perhaps the most important implication of cloning the PKD1 gene is that the primary defect in this common disease can now be studied. The author calls for research to gain a better understanding of how polycystin functions in health and disease, the molecules with which it interacts, what factors modify the disease phenotype, and the basic molecular mechanism by which cysts arise. Genetic linkage studies and renal (kidney) ultrasound scanning remain the investigations of choice in the diagnosis of patients with suspected ADPKD. 3 figures. 16 references.

- **Identification of Patients with Autosomal Dominant Polycystic Kidney Disease at Highest Risk for End-Stage Renal Disease**

Source: JASN. Journal of the American Society of Nephrology. 8(10): 1560-1547. October 1997.

Contact: Available from Williams and Wilkins. 428 E. Preston Street, Baltimore, MD 21202. (800) 638-6423.

Summary: This article reports on a study undertaken to identify which patients with autosomal dominant polycystic kidney disease (ADPKD) are at highest risk for end-stage renal disease (ESRD). In the study, survival analysis and risk ratio calculation for 1,215 patients with ADPKD were performed. Survival times were calculated as time to dialysis, transplantation, or death. Of the population studied, 388 patients entered ESRD and 205 patients died. ADPKD2 subjects had longer renal survival than ADPKD1 subjects (median survival 68 versus 53 years). Women had significantly better renal survival than men (56 versus 52 years). Subjects who were diagnosed before age 30 and those who developed hypertension before age 35 had worse renal survival than those subjects who were diagnosed after age 30 or those who remained normotensive after age 35, respectively. Similarly, those who had an episode of gross hematuria before age 30 had a worse renal outcome than those who did not. The authors conclude that, when therapeutic interventions become available for this disease, these populations with high risk ratios should be considered for such interventions. 10 figures. 2 tables. 23 references. (AA-M).

- **Autosomal Dominant Polycystic Kidney Disease**

  Source: American Family Physician. 53(3): 925-931. February 15, 1996.

  Summary: The author presents an overview of autosomal dominant polycystic kidney disease (ADPKD), one of the most commonly inherited diseases in the United States. Topics include a definition of ADPKD; genetic influence; symptoms and clinical presentation; pathology; complications and management including hypertension, hematuria, proteinuria, flank and abdominal pain, urinary tract infections, end-stage renal disease, renal calculi, renal cell carcinoma, vascular complications, liver disease, cardiac disease, gastrointestinal problems, and hematologic symptoms; dialysis in patients with ADPKD; renal transplantation in this population; research efforts for the treatment of ADPKD; and implications for patients and family members. 2 figures. 1 table. 23 references. (AA-M).

- **Polycystic Kidney Disease: Guidelines for Family Physicians**

  Source: American Family Physician. 53(3): 847-850. February 15, 1996.

  Summary: This editorial serves as an introduction to a companion article about autosomal dominant polycystic kidney disease (ADPKD). The author reminds readers that the outlook for patients with ADPKD has improved and discusses five basic points physicians should keep in mind when treating these patients. These points include understanding the genetic heterogeneity and marked phenotypic variability of ADPKD; distinguishing ADPKD from other renal cystic diseases; knowing why, when, and how to screen family members for the presence of the disease; detecting and treating conditions that may affect the outcome of ADPKD, notably hypertension; and promptly identifying problems that require specialized evaluation and treatment. 1 reference.

- **Dietary Protein Restriction, Blood Pressure Control, and the Progression of Polycystic Kidney Disease**

  Source: Journal of the American Society of Nephrology. 5(12): 2037-2047. June 1995.

  Contact: Available from Williams and Wilkins. 428 East Preston Street, Baltimore, MD 21202-3993. (800) 638-6423.

  Summary: In the Modification of Diet in Renal Disease Study, a followup (mean, 2.2 years) of 200 study participants with autosomal dominant polycystic kidney disease (ADPKD) was conducted to determine the effect of lowering protein intake and blood pressure on the rate of decline in glomerular filtration rate (GFR). This article reports on that study. The rate of decline was faster in participants with ADPKD than in persons with other diagnoses, reflecting, in part, faster disease progression in the ADPKD group. Baseline characteristics that predicted a faster rate of decline in GFR in persons with ADPKD were greater serum creatinine (independent of GFR), greater urinary protein excretion, higher mean arterial pressure (MAP), and younger age. Lower protein intake, but not prescription of the keto acid-amino acid supplement, was marginally associated with a slower progression of renal disease. 5 figures. 7 tables. 47 references.

- **Polycystic Kidney Disease 1 (PKD1) Gene Encodes a Novel Protein With Multiple Cell Recognition Domains**

  Source: Nature Genetics. 10(2): 151-159. June 1995.

  Contact: Available from Nature Genetics. Subscription Department, 345 Park Avenue South, New York, NY 10010. (212) 726-9200.

  Summary: Autosomal dominant polycystic kidney disease (ADPKD) is a frequent genetic disorder characterized by progressive cyst formation and enlargement, typically leading to end-stage renal disease (ESRD) by late middle age. In this article, the authors describe their work with characterization of the polycystic kidney disease 1 (PKD1) gene, noting that this work has been complicated by the genomic rearrangements on chromosome 16. They describe the use of an exon linking strategy, taking RNA from a cell line containing PKD1 but not the duplicate loci, to clone a cDNA sequence of the entire transcript. The predicted PKD1 protein, polycystin, is a glycoprotein with multiple transmembrane domains and a cytoplasmic C-tail. Their results indicate that polycystin is an integral membrane protein involved in cell-cell/matrix interactions. 8 figures. 2 tables. (AA-M).

Federally-Funded Research on Polycystic Kidney Disease

The U.S. Government supports a variety of research studies relating to polycystic kidney disease and associated conditions. These studies are tracked by the Office of Extramural Research at the National Institutes of Health.[16] CRISP (Computerized Retrieval of Information on Scientific

---

[16] Healthcare projects are funded by the National Institutes of Health (NIH), Substance Abuse and Mental Health Services (SAMHSA), Health Resources and Services Administration (HRSA), Food and Drug Administration (FDA), Centers for Disease Control

Projects) is a searchable database of federally-funded biomedical research projects conducted at universities, hospitals, and other institutions. Visit the site at **http://commons.cit.nih.gov/crisp3/CRISP.Generate_Ticket**. You can perform targeted searches by various criteria including geography, date, as well as topics related to polycystic kidney disease and related conditions.

For most of the studies, the agencies reporting into CRISP provide summaries or abstracts. As opposed to clinical trial research using patients, many federally-funded studies use animals or simulated models to explore polycystic kidney disease and related conditions. In some cases, therefore, it may be difficult to understand how some basic or fundamental research could eventually translate into medical practice. The following sample is typical of the type of information found when searching the CRISP database for polycystic kidney disease:

- **Project Title: A Model for Polycystic Kidney Disease in C Elegans**

  Principal Investigator & Institution: Barr, Maureen M.; None; University of Wisconsin Madison 500 Lincoln Dr Madison, Wi 53706

  Timing: Fiscal Year 2001; Project Start 1-MAY-2001; Project End 0-APR-2006

  Summary: (Applicant's Abstract): Autosomal Dominant Polycystic Kidney Disease (ADPKD) strikes 1 in 1000 individuals, often resulting in end-stage renal failure. Mutations in either PKD1 or PKD2 account for 95 percent of all cases. ADPKD1 and ADPKD2 are phenotypically indistinguishable, leading to the hypothesis that pathology is caused by defects in the same pathway. The cellular roles of the PKD 1 and PKD2 gene products (polycystin 1 and polycystin 2, respectively) still remain unknown. The powerful molecular genetic tools of the nematode Caenorhabditis elegans (C. Elegans)will enable us to address fundamental questions regarding polycystin function and physiological relevance of partner interactions. The C. elegans homologs of PKD1 and PKD2, LOV-1 and PKD-2, are coexpressed and colocalized in three types of male chemosensory neurons: the cephalic CEMs, the HOB hook neuron, and the ray neurons. Furthermore, lov-1 and pkd-2 are required in the male nervous system for the mating behaviors of response to hermaphrodite contact and location of the hermaphrodite vulva (Lov). The C. elegans homolog of Tg737 (a murine gene associated with Autosomal Recessive PKD) exhibits an expression pattern that partially overlaps with lov-1 and pkd-2 and maps closely to osm-5. osm-5 is also necessary for response and Lov behavior, suggesting that the three may

and Prevention (CDCP), Agency for Healthcare Research and Quality (AHRQ), and Office of Assistant Secretary of Health (OASH).

operate in the same cell. This proposal is designed to test the hypothesis that LOV-1, PKD-2, and possibly CeTg737 act in a common pathway. Experiments will explore several models of LOV-1, PKD-2, and CeTg737 function. Hypotheses include the following: CeTg737 may localize LOV-1 and PKD-2 to the cilia where LOV-1 and PKD-2 are required for function. Moreover, LOV-1 may be involved in transducing an extracellular signal via PKD-2 in the cilia, culminating in activation of an intracellular signaling pathway. Alternatively, LOV-1 and PKD-2 may be involved in the formation and maintenance of sensory cilia or the establishment and maintenance of neuronal cell polarity. A number of complementary studies are proposed to address the function of the C. elegans polycystins and CeTg737 in male mating behavior. Genetic and molecular interactions between lov-1, pkd-2, and CeTg737 will be explored. Cellular functions of the C. elegans polycystins will be ascertained. The function of CeTg737 in male sensory mating behaviors will be determined. New components in the LOV/PKD pathway will be isolated. These experiments will analyze LOV/PKD at the cellular, genetic, and molecular levels.

Website: http://commons.cit.nih.gov/crisp3/CRISP.Generate_Ticket

- **Project Title: Mechanisms of Aberrant EGF Receptor Sorting in Polycystic Kidney Disease**

Principal Investigator & Institution: Carlin, Cathleen R.; ; Case Western Reserve University 10900 Euclid Ave Cleveland, Oh 44106

Timing: Fiscal Year 2000

Summary: Formation of epithelial cell polarity is a fundamental process in embryonic development and organogenesis. Polarized epithelia in adult animals form a physical barrier between the host and external environment essential for homeostasis. Polarized epithelia maintain distinct apical (Ap) and basolateral (BL) membrane domains, by actively regulating membrane distribution of lipids and proteins as well as the sub- membranous cytoskeleton unique to each surface. Many questions remain about how membrane polarity is achieved, chief among them how Ap and BL proteins are packaged in distinct transport vesicles at the trans-Golgi- network (TGN). Sorting of BL proteins is mediated in part through recognition of distinct cytoplasmic sorting signals that also appear to regulate polarized sorting in endosomes. Although many BL sorting signals have common features, consensus motifs have not emerged, making it unclear whether all BL signals mediate transport by the same or different pathways. We propose to address this question by studying a novel autonomous Bl signal which we have identified in the EGF receptor (EGFR). This signal is located between residues K652 to

A674 in the EGFR juxta- membrane domain, and mediates BL transport of cytoplasmically truncated EGFRs and protein chimeras containing a luminal. This BL signal critical tyrosine and leucine residues and do not overlap any of the known EGFR endocytic signals, features that distinguish it from many other well- characterized BL sorting signals. Computer modeling suggests a propensity for this region to form an amphipathic helix, in contrast to other BL signals whose critical structure suggests a propensity for this region to form a amphipathic helix, in contrast to other BL signals whose critical structure in a beta-turn. This region also induce T654, a known substrate for protein kinase C, raising the possibility that its activity is regulated by phosphorylation. Immediate goals are to understand the mechanism by which this signal establishes and maintains EGFR' polarity. A long-term goal is to understand how genes which cause polycystic kidney disease alter this process, since non-polar EGFR expression is a common finding that renal cysts both in humans and animals disease models. The specific aims will: test the hypothesis that BL sorting of cytoplasmically truncated EGFRs is critically dependent on particular amino acids in the BL signal; test the hypothesis that residues K652 to A674 regulate BL transport of full-length EGFRs; test the hypothesis that residues K652 to A674 regulate polarized sorting in endosomes; and characterize elements of the EGFR sorting machinery by identifying proteins that interact with EGFR residues K652 to A674.

Website: http://commons.cit.nih.gov/crisp3/CRISP.Generate_Ticket

- **Project Title: Mouse Models of Polycystic Kidney Disease (PKD2)**

Principal Investigator & Institution: Somlo, Stefan; Associate Professor; Internal Medicine; Yale University New Haven, Ct 06520

Timing: Fiscal Year 2000; Project Start 5-JUN-1998; Project End 1-MAY-2003

Summary: (Adapted from the Applicant's Abstract): "The primary interest of our research is unraveling the pathogenesis of polycystic kidney disease. To this end, they have used positional cloning to identify the second gene for human autosomal dominant polycystic kidney disease (PKD2). The current proposal centers on the hypothesis that genetically altering the murine homologue of the PKD2 gene, Pkd2, will enable us to produce animal models whose phenotypes are faithful to those of human autosomal dominant polycystic kidney disease (ADPKD). They have produced a mouse line with a targeted mutation in which the first coding exon of Pkd2 has been disrupted. Mice heterozygous and homozygous for this allele develop polycystic kidneys and livers that recapitulate the human disease phenotype. The disease develops faster in homozygotes. They propose histopathological and functional characterization of the renal and extra-renal phenotypes of these mutant mouse lines as well as further analysis of the molecular consequences of the gene targeting event. This murine model of ADPKD has some residual polycystin-2 expression in the homozygous state. They propose to create a model in which exons 1, 2, and 3 of Pkd2 have been deleted. These null mice will provide a model system for studying the phenotype. In addition, they propose to introduce naturally occurring premature termination codons found in human families with ADPKD, into Pkd2. They will characterize the ensuing mouse phenotypes in heterozygous and homozygous mice and will characterize the functional consequences, at the level of the protein product, of these truncating mutations. Finally, they plan to study the effects of factors other than germ line mutation in Pkd2 on the occurrence and progression of the renal and extrarenal manifestations in mouse models of ADPKD. They will use marker assisted breeding strategies to produce congenic strains bearing mutations in Pkd2 on different genetic backgrounds. They will investigate the effects of defects in DNA mismatch repair on the progression of ADPKD by breeding Pkd2 mutations onto a MLH1-deficient mouse line."

Website: http://commons.cit.nih.gov/crisp3/CRISP.Generate_Ticket

- **Project Title: Pathophysiology of Recessive Polycystic Kidney Disease**

Principal Investigator & Institution: Avner, Ellis D.; Professor; Pediatrics; Case Western Reserve University 10900 Euclid Ave Cleveland, Oh 44106

Timing: Fiscal Year 2000; Project Start 0-SEP-1999; Project End 1-AUG-2004

Summary: OVERALL (Taken directly from the application) The overall objective for the development of an Interdisciplinary Center for Polycystic Kidney Disease Research at Case Western Reserve University (CWRU) is to attract a partnership of interdisciplinary research among investigators who will use complementary and integrated approaches to study the molecular and cellular pathophysiology of autosomal recessive polycystic kidney disease (ARPKD). ARPKD has an incidence of 1: 10,000 to 1: 40,000, has a mortality of 40-65% in the newborn period, and accounts for approximately 5% of all end-stage renal disease in children. Other than end-stage renal disease therapy and palliative measures designed to treat the complications of progressive portal hypertension, there is no known therapy for progressive renal cyst formation and enlargement or progressive biliary ectasia and fibrosis in ARPKD. Therefore the overall goal of the Center is to support scientific investigation directed at delineating the fundamental aspects of the disease process which will translate into the design of preventative and/or curative strategies for ARPKD. An ancillary objective of the Center is to attract new scientific expertise to the study of polycystic kidney disease. To achieve the stated objectives of the Center, the program involves a interdisciplinary research team drawn from the Departments of Pediatrics, Genetics, and Physiology & Biophysics at CWRU. The three Projects, three Cores, and two Pilot and Feasibility studies are scientifically integrated into an overall scheme which follows directly from current understanding of the molecular and cellular pathophysiology of ARPKD. Project 1, "Epithelial Growth Factor Mislocalization in ARPKD" focuses on a key process mediating abnormal epithelial cell proliferation. Project 2, "Altered Collecting Tubule Ion Transport in ARPKD" focuses on abnormalities in key ion transport processes which mediate altered tubular fluid secretion. Project 3, "Pharmacological and Genetic Therapy of ARPKD" is a translational project to develop therapeutic strategies which target key processes operative in the development and progression of disease. To support the scientific program, an Administrative Core will coordinate Center activities and specifically focus on maximizing scientific interactions of Center Investigators while monitoring and critically evaluating scientific process and encouraging new research in polycystic kidney disease-related areas. A Transgenic & Animal Resource Core will facilitate whole animal experimental approaches for all projects of the Center using state-of-the-art molecular genetic technology. A Cell Culture Core will provide and maintain primary cells and cell lines from human and murine control and cystic kidneys for the proposed studies. Though largely focused on the molecular and cellular pathophysiology of ARPKD, much of the basic knowledge and many of the treatment strategies developed by the Center will also have relevance to the study and treatment of autosomal dominant polycystic kidney disease.

Website: http://commons.cit.nih.gov/crisp3/CRISP.Generate_Ticket

- **Project Title: Polycystic Kidney Disease Gene of C. Elegans**

Principal Investigator & Institution: Buechner, Matthew J.; Assistant Professor; University of Kansas Medical Center Medical Center Kansas City, Ks 66103

Timing: Fiscal Year 2000; Project Start 0-SEP-1999; Project End 1-AUG-2004

Summary: (Taken directly from the application) Polycystic kidney disease (PKD) is a common genetic condition that results from the swelling of the lumen of the renal tubular epithelia; in addition, other tubular epithelia throughout the body, and in particular the liver, can exhibit similar deformations. The formation and maintenance of tubular diameter are poorly understood processes. Several cloned mammalian genes encode proteins essential for maintaining proper nephritic diameter and preventing cyst formation. Two proteins, termed polycystins, share a region of homology, and are both necessary for normal tubule structure, and prevention of an autosomal dominant PKD. A third protein, Tg737, prevents autosomal recessive PKD in mice. The biochemical functions of the polycystins is unclear; they may function together as an ion channel. Tg737 probably acts to bring proteins together in a complex, although the nature of those proteins is unknown. Close homologues to Polycystin 2 and Tg737 have been found by the genome project recently completed for the relatively simple creature, the nematode Caenorhabditis elegans. This worm is an attractive organism for studying the cellular function through the use of genetic techniques, and to discover the partners of these proteins in determining nephritic diameter. This application proposes: 1) To clone the CePKD-2 and CeTg737 genes from C elegans, and to determine the time and place of expression of these genes and their products during development; 2) To compare the function of the human and nematode PKD2 proteins through the construction of chimeric worm::human PKD-2 genes, and the production and analysis of transgenic nematodes containing these chimeric genes; 3) To create and examine the phenotype of a knockout mutant devoid of CeTg737 function, and to use genetic techniques to discover the proteins with which CeTg737 interacts. These experiments will elucidate the role of polycystin and Tg737 in maintaining tubule diameter, which will provide a major step towards understanding the causes of PKD.

Website: http://commons.cit.nih.gov/crisp3/CRISP.Generate_Ticket

- **Project Title: Caspases and Apoptosis in ADPKD**

    Principal Investigator & Institution: Edelstein, Charles L.; Associate Professor of Medicine; University of Colorado Hlth Sciences Ctr 4200 E 9Th Ave Denver, Co 80262

    Timing: Fiscal Year 2001; Project Start 1-APR-1985; Project End 0-JUN-2006

Summary: Autosomal Dominant Polycystic kidney Disease (ADPKD) is the most common life threatening hereditary disease in the USA and it accounts for about 5-10% of end-stage renal failure requiring dialysis and renal transplantation. Apoptosis in cells lining the cysts as well as in non-cystic is a characteristic feature of animal models of ADPKD as well as human ADPKD. Apoptosis is thought to play a role in both cyst formation and the loss of normal tubules and subsequent renal failure.

The central component of the apoptosis machinery is a novel family of cysteine proteases called caspases. Cell permeable caspase inhibitors have been widely used in animal studies in vivo to dramatically alter a variety of pathological processes. The effect of caspase inhibition on apoptosis, proliferation, cyst formation and renal failure in ADPKD forms the basis of this grant proposal. The overall hypothesis presented in this grant proposes that dysregulation of the balance between pro and anti-apoptotic Bcl-2 family proteins leads to activation of the "initiator" caspases 8 or 9 and the "executioner" caspase-3. Further, it is proposed that apoptosis precedes proliferation leading to cyst formation and that apoptotic loss of non-cystic renal tubules leads to renal failure. Complementary studies will be performed in Han:SPRD rats and Pkd2 mutant mice, which closely resemble human ADPKD. In Specific Aim #1 we shall describe the time course and localization of apoptosis and proliferation. Specific Aim #2 focuses on in vivo studies to determine whether caspase inhibitors will attenuate apoptosis, proliferation, cyst formation and renal failure. Caspase activity, protein and gene expression will be measured. Functional (serum urea and creatinine) and morphological (renal cyst size, proliferation and apoptosis) correlates will be documented. In Specific Aim #3,, the relationship between Bcl-2 gene family protein expression and caspase-3 activity will determined. The potential relevance of these studies to clinical ADPKD is substantial and the results should provide leads to altering the course of ADPKD. This is particularly true because of the current availability of cell permeable, non toxic caspase antagonists that are active in vivo.

Website: http://commons.cit.nih.gov/crisp3/CRISP.Generate_Ticket

- **Project Title: Channel Properties of Polycystin 2**

Principal Investigator & Institution: Ehrlich, Barbara E.; Professor; Yale University New Haven, Ct 06520

Timing: Fiscal Year 2000

Summary: This project examines the properties of a new class of intracellular Ca channel formed by polycystin-2. To date two major classes of Ca release channel have been identified: the ryanodine receptor (RyR) and the inositol 1,4,5-trisphosphate receptor (InsP3R). Most cells contain both types of channel, but the relative densities vary dramatically. The co-existence of a variety of intracellular channels is not surprising as cells need to respond to diverse stimuli with specific responses. The hypotheses to be tested are: 1) Polycystin-2 is a unique calcium- permeable channel in the endoplasmic reticular membrane. 2) The calcium channel formed by polycystin-2 is regulated by intracellular factors, including magnesium, eicosanoids, cAMP and polycystin-1. 3) specific regions of the protein can be divided into functional domains. These domains are based upon mutations found in polycystin-2 from subsets or individuals affected with autosomal dominant polycystic kidney disease (ADPKD). 4) Changes in channel activity of polycystin-2 will modify intracellular calcium signaling. The preliminary results presented here show for the first time that polycystin-2 makes a novel calcium permeable channel in the endoplasmic membrane. The experiments outlined in this project will investigate the functional properties of polycystin-2 at the single channel level and will correlate the channel properties with cell and organ function. The results to be obtained will identify regulatory factors that may determine the mechanism of action of polycystin-2 at a molecular level and may suggest useful tretments for individuals affected with polycystic kidney disease.

Website: http://commons.cit.nih.gov/crisp3/CRISP.Generate_Ticket

- **Project Title: Functional Analysis of Polycystin in Drosophila**

Principal Investigator & Institution: Lu, Xiangyi; University of Kansas Medical Center Medical Center Kansas City, Ks 66103

Timing: Fiscal Year 2000

Summary: (Taken directly from the application) Polycystic kidney disease (PKD) is a multigene disorder characterized by the growth of fluid-filled cysts, mainly in the kidney. Mutations in at least three genes, PKD1, PKD2 and PKD3, may give rise to the autosomal dominant form of PKD (ADPKD). Evidence suggests that the etiology of cyst initiation associated with PKD1 mutations results from two separate gene inactivation events. The first is an inherited mutation in one PKD1 allele; the second mutation arises in the normal allele during kidney development or maturation. We will test this "second hit" hypothesis as a mechanism for the onset of polycystic kidney disease by producing mice containing both a primary mutation in Pkd1 and a conditional second-hit mutation that can be induced somatically in the other murine Pkd1 allele. These mice will be analyzed for phenotypes associated with ADPKD. Additionally, the combination of mutations will test the Pkd1 missense mutation (Project 3) in a more physiologically relevant model. Finally, the long-range goal of this project is to generate an animal model in which the development of renal, hepatic and other pathophysiology associated with polycystic kidney disease can be analyzed and understood and in which modes of treatment can be tested.

Website: http://commons.cit.nih.gov/crisp3/CRISP.Generate_Ticket

- **Project Title: Kansas Interdisciplinary Center for PKD Research**

Principal Investigator & Institution: Grantham, Jared J.; Distinguished Professor; Biochemistry; University of Kansas Medical Center Medical Center Kansas City, Ks 66103

Timing: Fiscal Year 2000; Project Start 0-SEP-1999; Project End 1-AUG-2004

Summary: OVERALL (Taken directly from the application) Polycystic kidney disease is observed throughout the animal kingdom. In humans it frequently leads to renal failure. It is widely believed that the destructive consequences of this group of diseases rest in the development of cysts within renal tubule segments and their growth to enormous size. The Kansas Interdisciplinary Center for PKD Research will build-on a rich history of basic and clinical polycystic kidney disease research at this site to address important questions about the molecular and cellular pathogenesis of cyst development and growth. The theme of this Center application is 'Polycystin and signal transduction in polycystic kidney disease". Four established PKD investigators and one established researcher new to this field are Principal Investigators of five research projects. An administrative Core will include a pilot and feasibility study by an established molecular biologist who is new to the field. All of the projects are explicitly linked to the study of polycystic kidney disease and range from studies of polycystin mutations in lower organisms to the molecular mechanisms by which cysts develop and progressively enlarge in mammals. Lower animals serve as a road map to functions that are highly conserved in the biologic kingdom. Project 1 will determine the patterns of expression and comparative functions of two cyst-forming genes, CePKD-2 and CeTg737, in C. elegans. Project 2 will establish a model of polycystic kidney disease in Drosophila in order to reconstruct the network of molecular events in the PKD1/PKD2 mediated pathway. Project 3 will test the hypothesis that PKD1 functions as a G-protein coupled receptor that when mutated disturbs early embryological development and the development of the kidney and other organ systems. Project 4 will test the hypothesis that polycystin-1 regulates signal transduction pathways that modulate the activity of glucocorticoid receptor using the glucocorticoid-induced expression of the renal glutathione S-transferase Ya gene as a model system. Project 5 will test the hypothesis that in ADPKD, renal cyst enlargement is accelerated by elevated levels of intracellular cyclic AMP that, through the activation of protein kinase A, stimulates other cellular mechanisms, most notably the ERK/MAP kinase pathway. Project 6 will test the "second hit" hypothesis as a mechanism for the onset of polycystic kidney disease by producing mice containing both a primary mutation in PKD 1 and an inducible second-hit somatic mutation in the other allele. The long term goal is for this research to contribute to novel treatments to slow or arrest the progression of polycystic kidney disorders.

Website: http://commons.cit.nih.gov/crisp3/CRISP.Generate_Ticket

- **Project Title: Modifier Genes in Autosomal Dominant Polycystic Kidney**

Principal Investigator & Institution: Fain, Pamela R.; Associate Professor; University of Colorado Hlth Sciences Ctr 4200 E 9Th Ave Denver, Co 80262

Timing: Fiscal Year 2001; Project Start 1-APR-1985; Project End 0-JUN-2006

Summary: There is extreme variability in the expression of ADPKD both between and within families. The factors contributing to these differences are largely unknown, but could be used to predict and potentially alter the clinical outcome of PKD mutations. The between-family variability could be due to locus heterogeneity, to allelic heterogeneity for mutations or wild-type alleles, and/or modifier genes. The within-family variability cannot be explained by either locus heterogeneity or by allelic heterogeneity for mutations, but could be due to allelic heterogeneity for wild-type PKD alleles or modifier genes. This study will use a large collection of clinically well-characterized ADPKD families to determine the effects of wild-type PKD alleles and modifier genes on phenotypic expression. Evidence supporting a 2-hit model of cystogenesis involving a somatic mutation in the wild-type and a distinct pattern of familial correlations for phenotypes relating to the timing and development of cysts, suggest a model in which different wild-type PKD alleles are associated with different somatic mutation rates. The model will be tested in Specific Aim 1 by determining if siblings who inherit the same wild-type PKD allele are more similar than siblings who inherit a different wild-type PKD allele. If so, association studies will be used to identify the specific wild-type PKD allele(s) that have a high somatic mutation rate(s). The pattern of familial correlations for other clinically-relevant ADPKD-related phenotypes, such as creatinine clearance, age at ESRD, and hypertension is consistent with the effects of modifier genes. However, the number of candidate modifier genes among known genes is very large; and one or more as yet unidentified genes could also be involved. Therefore, in Specific Aim 2, a genome screen for linkage will be used to identify positional candidate modifier genes, focusing initially on a subset of the most highly discordant families, followed by replication in families with severe phenotypes. Additional markers in regions where significant linkage is found in both samples will then be typed in all families in order to pinpoint the specific modifier gene(s). A final analysis will be performed to estimate the relative influence of different sources of phenotypic variability, and to investigate the genetic and environmental correlations among different phenotypes.

Website: http://commons.cit.nih.gov/crisp3/CRISP.Generate_Ticket

- **Project Title: Molecular Characterization of the JCPK/BPK Locus**

Principal Investigator & Institution: Bryda, Elizabeth C.; Micro/Immunol/Molec Genetics; Marshall University 400 Hal Greer Blvd Huntington, Wv 25701

Timing: Fiscal Year 2000; Project Start 5-MAR-1999; Project End 9-FEB-2004

Summary: (Adapted from Investigator's Abstract): The broad long-term objective of this proposal is to study the genetics of a mouse model for polycystic kidney disease to better understand renal cystogenesis. The specific aims for this proposal are to isolate and characterize the mouse jcpk/bpk gene and its human homologue. When inherited in an autosomal recessive manner, the mouse jcpk gene causes a severe form of early onset polycystic kidney disease (PKD) accompanied by a number of extrarenal effects. The jcpk model is unique from other mouse PKD models and has a phenotype with characteristics resembling both the dominant and recessive forms of PKD in humans. Recent studies have indicated that jcpk and another mouse PKD-causing mutation, bpk, are allelic, despite the different kidney disease phenotypes produced by each. Additionally, jcpk/bpk is a candidate for a locus that modifies the expression of a separate and distinct PKD caused by the jck gene. It is believed that modifying loci play an important role in human PKD based on highly variable intra familial clinical presentation and course of disease. In this grant application, we propose to identify both the mouse jcpk/bpk gene and its human homologue using molecular genetic techniques. The specific aims of this proposal are 1) to physically map the jcpk gene, 2) to isolate and characterize the jcpk/bpk gene and, 3) to isolate the human homologue of the mouse jcpk/bpk gene. GRANT=R01DK54741 (Adapted from Investigator's Abstract): Cytosolic phospholipase A2 (cPLA2) has been implicated in cell injury, however, the mechanisms by which cPLA2 acts are unknown. cPLA2 localizes to an intranuclear site in response to serum deprivation resulting in cell death. Two novel nuclear cPLA2-interacting proteins have been isolated. These cPLA2-interactors are homologous to yeast silencing genes, SIR2 and SAS2/SAS3. One of these interacting proteins, PLIP, (for Phospholipase A2-interacting protein), has an amino acid sequence containing a recently described MYST domain. The MYST domain is made up of an atypical C2HC zinc finger and a signature acetyltransferase sequence. The presence of this domain and homologies of PLIP to yeast drosophila and mammalian proteins suggest a potential role in transcriptional regulation for PLIP and thus cPLA2. The expression of PLIP in renal mesangial cells markedly enhances cell injury due to both serum deprivation and TNFalpha. It is likely that an intranuclear complex containing cPLA2 and the two interactor proteins mediates the mesangial cell response to TNFalpha and to serum deprivation. The first aim of this proposal is to examine mechanisms by which PLIP modulates cPLA2 activity and contributes to mesangial cell susceptibility to injury. The second specific aim is to characterize the second clone 46, to identify its role in cPLA2 regulation, and to determine its role, if any, in cell susceptibility to injury. To achieve these aims, basic techniques in molecular biology and cellular and lipid biochemistry will be used, specifically including site directed mutagenesis and an adenoviral expression system. Transfected constructs encoding a peroxosomal proliferator activated receptor (PPAR) and containing a reporter gene driven by a PPAR response element will be used for a functional readout of intranuclear arachidonic acid release. The completion of this proposal will greatly enhance our understanding of the role and regulation of cPLA2 in cell injury.

Website: http://commons.cit.nih.gov/crisp3/CRISP.Generate_Ticket

- **Project Title: Molecular Pathology of Polycyrstic Kidney Disease**

Principal Investigator & Institution: Zhou, Jing; Associate Professor; Brigham and Women's Hospital 75 Francis St Boston, Ma 02115

Timing: Fiscal Year 2000; Project Start 1-JAN-1989; Project End 1-MAR-2004

Summary: (Verbatim from Investigator's Abstract): Polycystic kidney disease comprises a group of genetic disorders caused by mutations in at least 5 genetically distinct genes. The most common form of PKD, autosomal dominant polycystic kidney disease (ADPKD), is one of the most common monogenic genetic diseases (PDPKD) of man, affecting about 1 in 1,000 individuals. ADPKD leads to cystic replacement of renal tissue and progressive renal failure, requiring renal replacement therapy in half of the cases by age 50. It is a systemic disease involving not only the kidney but also the liver, pancreas, arteries and heart. Polycystins comprise a new class of membrane-spanning proteins. To date, four polycystins, encoded by four genetically distinct genes, have been identified. Polycystins -1, and -2, are mutated in autosomal dominant polycystic kidney disease (ADPKD). Polycystins-REJ and -L, which are mostly closely related to polycystin -1 and -2, respectively, are not yet implicated in disease states. The polycystin family can be divided into polycystin-1 (PC1)-like and polycystin-2(PC2)-like subgroups. Both PC2-like proteins (polycystins-2 and -L) share structural homology with cation channels such as those of the transient receptor potential (TRP) and voltage-gated Ca2+, Na+ and K+ channel families. On the other hand, both PC1-like molecules, polycystins-1 and -REJ, share significant domain and sequence homology to a putative ion channel regulator (receptor for egg jelly) in sea urchins. The object of this renewal proposal is to extend the functional studies of polycystin -1 and polycystin-L. Three main lines of investigation will be pursued. First, further characterization of two previously identified potential binding partners of polycystin-1, and continue to search for polycystin-1 ligands. Second, extending the recent studies that show that polycystin-L has channel properties and determine whether other polycystins (1 and 2) modulate these properties. Lastly, complement these biochemical and biophysical studies with gene targeting experiments to elucidate the biological functions of polycystin-L in vivo.

Website: http://commons.cit.nih.gov/crisp3/CRISP.Generate_Ticket

- **Project Title: Redox, Acid/Base, and Pathogenesis of ADPKD**

Principal Investigator & Institution: Torres, Vicente E.; Chairman; Mayo Clinic Rochester 200 1St St Sw Rochester, Mn 55905

Timing: Fiscal Year 2000; Project Start 0-SEP-1995; Project End 1-AUG-2003

Summary: (Verbatim from Investigator's Abstract): In the previous grant cycle, we have demonstrated that the development of polycystic kidney disease in the Han:SPRD rat is accompanied by abnormalities in redox metabolism, that the acid content of the diet and/or experimental modifications of the redox state have profound effects on renal cystogenesis in Han:SPRD rats and pcy mice and on renal carcinogenesis in Eker rats, and that extracellular acidification increases the production of oxidant species and the rate of somatic mutations in cultured tubular epithelial cells. We hypothesize that oxidative stress resulting from acid administration, glutathione depletion, genetically determined deficiencies of CuZn superoxide dismutase (SOD1), Mn superoxide dismutase (SOD2) or selenium dependent cellular glutathione peroxidase (GPX1), or a combination of these factors will promote cystogenesis in Pkd1 del34/+ and Pkd2 -/+ mice by increasing the rate of mutation of the wild type Pkd1 and Pkd2 genes. Conversely we hypothesize that base administration will reduce the rate of intragenic homologous recombination between tandemly repeated portions of the wild-type and mutant exons 1 within the WS25 allele and will reduce the severity of polycystic kidney disease in compound heterozygous Pkd2 -/WS25 mice. Finally, we hypothesize that the generation of oxidant species in tubular epithelial cells in response to acidification or glutathione depletion is a lipid peroxyl or alkoxyl radical and that the rate of production of this radical in response to acidification or glutathione depletion in vitro and in vivo depends on the cell fatty acid composition and affects the development of polycystic kidney disease. Measurements of tissue levels of glutathione and activities of SOD1, SOD2, and GPX1 will be performed to control for the experimental conditions. The severity of the polycystic kidney disease will be assessed by histomorphometric analysis and determinations of plasma creatinine and urea. Immunohistology, together with laser capture microdissection of individual cyst cell populations, PCR amplification, and DNA sequencing will be used to assess the molecular mechanism of cyst formation. The effect of cell fatty acid composition on the generation of oxidant species, lipid peroxyl and alkoxyl radicals, mutagenesis and cystogenesis will be studied in cell culture systems using a DCF fluorometric assay, electron paramagnetic resonance, and an SV40-based shuttle vector containing suppressor tyrosyl tRNA as a target for mutagenesis, as well as in Pkd1 -/+ and Pkd2 -/+ mice. The main thrust of the proposed studies is directed towards the identification of pathogenetic mechanisms than can be subject to preventive and therapeutic interventions.

Website: http://commons.cit.nih.gov/crisp3/CRISP.Generate_Ticket

- **Project Title: Renal Cystic Maldevelopment**

Principal Investigator & Institution: Drummond, Iain; ; Massachusetts General Hospital 55 Fruit St Boston, Ma 02114

Timing: Fiscal Year 2000

Summary: Polycystic kidney disease is a complex disorder which can result from a variety of gene mutations as well as from environmental insults. Developmental or cellular defects in epithelia caused by cystic mutations are often obscured by compensatory tissue responses, making it difficult to define the primary cause of cystic disease. Despite recent advances in cloning the genes responsible for the majority of polycystic kidney disease (PKD1, PKD2), the function of these genes in normal epithelia remains unknown. The goal of this proposal is to take advantage of the zebrafish as a genetic and developmental system to 1) explore the primary defects in the pronephros caused by cystic mutations in the absence of glomerular filtration, 2) clone and further characterize the zebrafish PKD1 homolog, 3) using a candidate gene approach screen for mutations in zfPKD1 in an existing set of pronephric cyst mutants, and 4) explore the potentially dominant-negative or constitutively active function and of the C-terminal cytoplasmic tail of PKD1 by expressing it in vivo in the context of zebrafish development. This study will identify initial defects associated with cystic mutations and in so doing, help focus the development of therapies on the primary causes of cystic disease. In addition, we will identify cellular and tissue responses which may modify the rate of disease progression or age of onset. The ability to study the PKD1 gene in a system which lends itself to genetic linkage studies, direct observation of development, and embryonic manipulation makes possible an analysis of the role of PKD1 in early development and the onset of cyst formation, determination of cell-autonomous or non cell-autonomous functions of PKD1, and the identification of evolutionarily conserved and functionally important domains of PKD1. It is our hope that the availability of a simple and accessible cystic disease model will help identify novel targets for therapeutic interventions and speed the development treatments for polycystic kidney disease.

Website: http://commons.cit.nih.gov/crisp3/CRISP.Generate_Ticket

- **Project Title: The Role of TGF-Alpha in the Pathogenesis of ARPKD**

Principal Investigator & Institution: Dell, Katherine M.; Pediatrics; Case Western Reserve University 10900 Euclid Ave Cleveland, Oh 44106

Timing: Fiscal Year 2001; Project Start 1-JUL-2001; Project End 0-JUN-2006

Summary: (adapted from the application) Autosomal recessive polycystic kidney disease (ARPKD) is an inherited kidney disorder characterized by massive kidney enlargement and hepatic fibrosis. Progression to end-stage renal disease is usually inevitable, often in the first years of life. A growing body of literature has established a key role for the epidermal growth factor receptor (EGFR) in the pathogenesis of abnormal cell proliferation and cyst expansion. In contrast, the expression, regulation, and function of the EGFR ligands have not been studied systematically in these diseases. Published data demonstrate that the EGFR ligand, transforming growth factor-alpha (TGF-alpha), is overexpressed in cystic tissues and cells and transgenic mice that overexpress TGF-alpha develop renal cysts. Using TGF-alpha as a paradigm, the proposed research will examine the physiologic effects of ligand upregulation and identify factors that contribute to EGFR ligand overexpression in ARPKD. The central hypothesis is that aberrant EGFR ligand expression is a common feature modulating the cellular pathophysiology of PKD. The specific aims of the project are: 1. To examine the physiologic effects of TGF-alpha upregulation in cyst formation and enlargement and to identify specific factors mediating TGF-alpha upregulation. Specific hypothesis to be tested include: a) TGF-alpha upregulation results in increased production of itself (auto-induction) and other EGFR ligands (cross-induction); b) secreted, not membrane-bound TGF-alpha, is the more important biologically-active moiety in ARPKD; c) TGF-alpha regulates EGFR expression by direct effects on EGFR mRNA transcription and stability; and d) abnormal expression of AP-2 and VHL, factors known to regulate TGF-alpha expression, mediate increased TGF-alpha expression in ARPKD. Primary and immortalized collecting tubule (CT) cell lines derived from cystic bpk mice (a murine model of ARPKD) and noncystic littermates will be used to assess the in vitro effects of exogenous TGF-alpha administration, TGF-alpha overexpression, and TGF-alpha/EGFR interactions. AP-2 and VHL protein and mRNA expression in cystic and control tissues and cells will be determined, and the role of each protein in TGF-alpha regulation assessed. 2. To determine the in vivo effects of blocking TGF-alpha production on disease progression in ARPKD. The hypothesis to be tested is that TGF-alpha has a key role in the pathogenesis of ARPKD. This will be tested by breeding the bpk mouse with a TGF-alpha knockout mouse and assessing the impact on disease progression and expression of EGFR and other EGFR ligands. These studies will provide new insights into the biology of EGFR ligands in ARPKD. Although the proposed research focuses on ARPKD, insights provided by these studies may contribute to a broader understanding of autosomal dominant polycystic kidney disease (ADPKD) as well.

Website: http://commons.cit.nih.gov/crisp3/CRISP.Generate_Ticket

E-Journals: PubMed Central[17]

PubMed Central (PMC) is a digital archive of life sciences journal literature developed and managed by the National Center for Biotechnology Information (NCBI) at the U.S. National Library of Medicine (NLM).[18] Access to this growing archive of e-journals is free and unrestricted.[19] To search, go to **http://www.pubmedcentral.nih.gov/index.html#search**, and type "polycystic kidney disease" (or synonyms) into the search box. This search

[17] Adapted from the National Library of Medicine:
http://www.pubmedcentral.nih.gov/about/intro.html.
[18] With PubMed Central, NCBI is taking the lead in preservation and maintenance of open access to electronic literature, just as NLM has done for decades with printed biomedical literature. PubMed Central aims to become a world-class library of the digital age.
[19] The value of PubMed Central, in addition to its role as an archive, lies the availability of data from diverse sources stored in a common format in a single repository. Many journals already have online publishing operations, and there is a growing tendency to publish material online only, to the exclusion of print.

gives you access to full-text articles. The following is a sample of items found for polycystic kidney disease in the PubMed Central database:

- **Abnormal Sodium Pump Distribution During Renal Tubulogenesis in Congenital Murine Polycystic Kidney Disease** by ED Avner, WE Sweeney, Jr, and WJ Nelson; 1992 August 15
  http://www.pubmedcentral.nih.gov/articlerender.fcgi?rendertype=abstract&artid=49727

- **Commentary:Polycystic kidney disease: In danger of being X-rated?** by Jared J. Grantham and James P. Calvet; 2001 January 30
  http://www.pubmedcentral.nih.gov/articlerender.fcgi?artid=33367

- **CpG Island in the Region of an Autosomal Dominant Polycystic Kidney Disease Locus Defines the 5' End of a Gene Encoding a Putative Proton Channel** by GAJ Gillespie, S Somlo, GG Germino, D Weinstat-Saslow, and ST Reeders; 1991 May 15
  http://www.pubmedcentral.nih.gov/articlerender.fcgi?rendertype=abstract&artid=51644

- **From the Cover:Polycystin-2, the protein mutated in autosomal dominant polycystic kidney disease (ADPKD), is a Ca2 +-permeable nonselective cation channel** by Silvia Gonzalez-Perrett, Keetae Kim, Cristina Ibarra, Alicia E. Damiano, Elsa Zotta, Marisa Batelli, Peter C. Harris, Ignacio L. Reisin, M. Amin Arnaout, and Horacio F. Cantiello; 2001 January 30
  http://www.pubmedcentral.nih.gov/articlerender.fcgi?artid=14729

- **Mutations in a NIMA-related kinase gene, Nek1, cause pleiotropic effects including a progressive polycystic kidney disease in mice** by Poornima Upadhya, Edward H. Birkenmeier, Connie S. Birkenmeier, and Jane E. Barker; 2000 January 4
  http://www.pubmedcentral.nih.gov/articlerender.fcgi?artid=26643

- **Polycystin, the Polycystic Kidney Disease 1 Protein, is Expressed by Epithelial Cells in Fetal, Adult, and Polycystic Kidney** by CJ Ward, H Turley, ACM Ong, M Comley, S Biddolph, R Chetty, PJ Ratcliffe, K Gatter, and PC Harris; 1996 February 20
  http://www.pubmedcentral.nih.gov/articlerender.fcgi?rendertype=abstract&artid=39973

- **Targeted Disruption of Bcl-2[alpha][beta] in Mice: Occurrence of Gray Hair, Polycystic Kidney Disease, and Lymphocytopenia** by K Nakayama, K Nakayama, I Negishi, K Kuida, H Sawa, and DY Loh; 1994 April 26
  http://www.pubmedcentral.nih.gov/articlerender.fcgi?rendertype=abstract&artid=43649

- **The polycystic kidney disease protein PKD2 interacts with Hax-1, a protein associated with the actin cytoskeleton** by Anna Rachel Gallagher, Anna Cedzich, Norbert Gretz, Stefan Somlo, and Ralph Witzgall; 2000 April 11
  http://www.pubmedcentral.nih.gov/articlerender.fcgi?artid=18134

The National Library of Medicine: PubMed

One of the quickest and most comprehensive ways to find academic studies in both English and other languages is to use PubMed, maintained by the National Library of Medicine. The advantage of PubMed over previously mentioned sources is that it covers a greater number of domestic and foreign references. It is also free to the public.[20] If the publisher has a Web site that offers full text of its journals, PubMed will provide links to that site, as well as to sites offering other related data. User registration, a subscription fee, or some other type of fee may be required to access the full text of articles in some journals.

To generate your own bibliography of studies dealing with polycystic kidney disease, simply go to the PubMed Web site at **www.ncbi.nlm.nih.gov/pubmed**. Type "polycystic kidney disease" (or synonyms) into the search box, and click "Go." The following is the type of output you can expect from PubMed for "polycystic kidney disease" (hyperlinks lead to article summaries):

- **Modification of polycystic kidney disease and fatty acid status by soy protein diet.**
  Author(s): Ogborn MR, Nitschmann E, Weiler HA, Bankovic-Calic N.
  Source: Kidney International. 2000 January; 57(1): 159-66.
  http://www.ncbi.nlm.nih.gov:80/entrez/query.fcgi?cmd=Retrieve&db=PubMed&list_uids=10620197&dopt=Abstract

- **Pain management in polycystic kidney disease.**
  Author(s): Bajwa ZH, Gupta S, Warfield CA, Steinman TI.

---

[20] PubMed was developed by the National Center for Biotechnology Information (NCBI) at the National Library of Medicine (NLM) at the National Institutes of Health (NIH). The PubMed database was developed in conjunction with publishers of biomedical literature as a search tool for accessing literature citations and linking to full-text journal articles at Web sites of participating publishers. Publishers that participate in PubMed supply NLM with their citations electronically prior to or at the time of publication.

Source: Kidney International. 2001 November; 60(5): 1631-44. Review.
http://www.ncbi.nlm.nih.gov:80/entrez/query.fcgi?cmd=Retrieve&db=
PubMed&list_uids=11703580&dopt=Abstract

Vocabulary Builder

Aberrant: Wandering or deviating from the usual or normal course. [EU]

Adenosine: A nucleoside that is composed of adenine and d-ribose. Adenosine or adenosine derivatives play many important biological roles in addition to being components of DNA and RNA. Adenosine itself is a neurotransmitter. [NIH]

Alleles: Mutually exclusive forms of the same gene, occupying the same locus on homologous chromosomes, and governing the same biochemical and developmental process. [NIH]

Arteries: The vessels carrying blood away from the heart. [NIH]

Assay: Determination of the amount of a particular constituent of a mixture, or of the biological or pharmacological potency of a drug. [EU]

Atypical: Irregular; not conformable to the type; in microbiology, applied specifically to strains of unusual type. [EU]

Biochemical: Relating to biochemistry; characterized by, produced by, or involving chemical reactions in living organisms. [EU]

Caenorhabditis: A genus of small free-living nematodes. Two species, caenorhabditis elegans and C. briggsae are much used in studies of genetics, development, aging, muscle chemistry, and neuroanatomy. [NIH]

Calculi: An abnormal concretion occurring mostly in the urinary and biliary tracts, usually composed of mineral salts. Also called stones. [NIH]

Carbohydrate: An aldehyde or ketone derivative of a polyhydric alcohol, particularly of the pentahydric and hexahydric alcohols. They are so named because the hydrogen and oxygen are usually in the proportion to form water, $(CH2O)n$. The most important carbohydrates are the starches, sugars, celluloses, and gums. They are classified into mono-, di-, tri-, poly- and heterosaccharides. [EU]

Carcinoma: A malignant new growth made up of epithelial cells tending to infiltrate the surrounding tissues and give rise to metastases. [EU]

Caspases: A family of intracellular cysteine endopeptidases. They play a key role in inflammation and mammalian apoptosis. They are specific for aspartic acid at the P1 position. They are divided into two classes based on the lengths of their N-terminal prodomains. Caspases-1,-2,-4,-5,-8, and -10 have long prodomains and -3,-6,-7,-9 have short prodomains. EC 3.4.22.-. [NIH]

Chimera: An individual that contains cell populations derived from different zygotes. [NIH]

Cyclic: Pertaining to or occurring in a cycle or cycles; the term is applied to chemical compounds that contain a ring of atoms in the nucleus. [EU]

Cysteine: A thiol-containing non-essential amino acid that is oxidized to form cystine. [NIH]

Cytoskeleton: The network of filaments, tubules, and interconnecting filamentous bridges which give shape, structure, and organization to the cytoplasm. [NIH]

Drosophila: A genus of small, two-winged flies containing approximately 900 described species. These organisms are the most extensively studied of all genera from the standpoint of genetics and cytology. [NIH]

Endoscopy: Visual inspection of any cavity of the body by means of an endoscope. [EU]

Endosomes: Cytoplasmic vesicles formed when coated vesicles shed their clathrin coat. Endosomes internalize macromolecules bound by receptors on the cell surface. [NIH]

Epidermal: Pertaining to or resembling epidermis. Called also epidermic or epidermoid. [EU]

Erythropoietin: Glycoprotein hormone, secreted chiefly by the kidney in the adult and the liver in the fetus, that acts on erythroid stem cells of the bone marrow to stimulate proliferation and differentiation. [NIH]

Exogenous: Developed or originating outside the organism, as exogenous disease. [EU]

Exons: Coding regions of messenger RNA included in the genetic transcript which survive the processing of RNA in cell nuclei to become part of a spliced messenger of structural RNA in the cytoplasm. They include joining and diversity exons of immunoglobulin genes. [NIH]

Filtration: The passage of a liquid through a filter, accomplished by gravity, pressure, or vacuum (suction). [EU]

Homeostasis: A tendency to stability in the normal body states (internal environment) of the organism. It is achieved by a system of control mechanisms activated by negative feedback; e.g. a high level of carbon dioxide in extracellular fluid triggers increased pulmonary ventilation, which in turn causes a decrease in carbon dioxide concentration. [EU]

Homologous: Corresponding in structure, position, origin, etc., as (a) the feathers of a bird and the scales of a fish, (b) antigen and its specific antibody, (c) allelic chromosomes. [EU]

Homozygote: An individual in which both alleles at a given locus are identical. [NIH]

Induction: The act or process of inducing or causing to occur, especially the production of a specific morphogenetic effect in the developing embryo through the influence of evocators or organizers, or the production of anaesthesia or unconsciousness by use of appropriate agents. [EU]

Invasive: 1. having the quality of invasiveness. 2. involving puncture or incision of the skin or insertion of an instrument or foreign material into the body; said of diagnostic techniques. [EU]

Leucine: An essential branched-chain amino acid important for hemoglobin formation. [NIH]

Lipid: Any of a heterogeneous group of flats and fatlike substances characterized by being water-insoluble and being extractable by nonpolar (or fat) solvents such as alcohol, ether, chloroform, benzene, etc. All contain as a major constituent aliphatic hydrocarbons. The lipids, which are easily stored in the body, serve as a source of fuel, are an important constituent of cell structure, and serve other biological functions. Lipids may be considered to include fatty acids, neutral fats, waxes, and steroids. Compound lipids comprise the glycolipids, lipoproteins, and phospholipids. [EU]

Lithotripsy: The destruction of a calculus of the kidney, ureter, bladder, or gallbladder by physical forces, including crushing with a lithotriptor through a catheter. Focused percutaneous ultrasound and focused hydraulic shock waves may be used without surgery. Lithotripsy does not include the dissolving of stones by acids or litholysis. Lithotripsy by laser is lithotripsy, laser. [NIH]

Localization: 1. the determination of the site or place of any process or lesion. 2. restriction to a circumscribed or limited area. 3. prelocalization. [EU]

Lumen: The cavity or channel within a tube or tubular organ. [EU]

Malformation: A morphologic defect resulting from an intrinsically abnormal developmental process. [EU]

Membrane: A thin layer of tissue which covers a surface, lines a cavity or divides a space or organ. [EU]

Mutagenesis: Process of generating genetic mutations. It may occur spontaneously or be induced by mutagens. [NIH]

Nephrology: A subspecialty of internal medicine concerned with the anatomy, physiology, and pathology of the kidney. [NIH]

Neurons: The basic cellular units of nervous tissue. Each neuron consists of a body, an axon, and dendrites. Their purpose is to receive, conduct, and transmit impulses in the nervous system. [NIH]

Normotensive: 1. characterized by normal tone, tension, or pressure, as by normal blood pressure. 2. a person with normal blood pressure. [EU]

Paclitaxel: Antineoplastic agent isolated from the bark of the Pacific yew tree, Taxus brevifolia. Paclitaxel stabilizes microtubules in their polymerized form and thus mimics the action of the proto-oncogene proteins C-MOS. [NIH]

Palliative: 1. affording relief, but not cure. 2. an alleviating medicine. [EU]

Pediatrics: A medical specialty concerned with maintaining health and providing medical care to children from birth to adolescence. [NIH]

Percutaneous: Performed through the skin, as injection of radiopacque material in radiological examination, or the removal of tissue for biopsy accomplished by a needle. [EU]

Peroxidase: A hemeprotein from leukocytes. Deficiency of this enzyme leads to a hereditary disorder coupled with disseminated moniliasis. It catalyzes the conversion of a donor and peroxide to an oxidized donor and water. EC 1.11.1.7. [NIH]

Phenotype: The outward appearance of the individual. It is the product of interactions between genes and between the genotype and the environment. This includes the killer phenotype, characteristic of yeasts. [NIH]

Phosphorylation: The introduction of a phosphoryl group into a compound through the formation of an ester bond between the compound and a phosphorus moiety. [NIH]

Protease: Proteinase (= any enzyme that catalyses the splitting of interior peptide bonds in a protein). [EU]

Proteins: Polymers of amino acids linked by peptide bonds. The specific sequence of amino acids determines the shape and function of the protein. [NIH]

Receptor: 1. a molecular structure within a cell or on the surface characterized by (1) selective binding of a specific substance and (2) a specific physiologic effect that accompanies the binding, e.g., cell-surface receptors for peptide hormones, neurotransmitters, antigens, complement fragments, and immunoglobulins and cytoplasmic receptors for steroid hormones. 2. a sensory nerve terminal that responds to stimuli of various kinds. [EU]

Renin: An enzyme of the hydrolase class that catalyses cleavage of the leucine-leucine bond in angiotensin to generate angiotensin. 1. The enzyme is synthesized as inactive prorenin in the kidney and released into the blood in the active form in response to various metabolic stimuli. Not to be confused with rennin (chymosin). [EU]

Retrograde: 1. moving backward or against the usual direction of flow. 2. degenerating, deteriorating, or catabolic. [EU]

Ryanodine: Insecticidal alkaloid isolated from Ryania speciosa; proposed as a myocardial depressant. [NIH]

Sclerosis: A induration, or hardening; especially hardening of a part from inflammation and in diseases of the interstitial substance. The term is used chiefly for such a hardening of the nervous system due to hyperplasia of the connective tissue or to designate hardening of the blood vessels. [EU]

Secretion: 1. the process of elaborating a specific product as a result of the activity of a gland; this activity may range from separating a specific substance of the blood to the elaboration of a new chemical substance. 2. any substance produced by secretion. [EU]

Selenium: An element with the atomic symbol Se, atomic number 34, and atomic weight 78.96. It is an essential micronutrient for mammals and other animals but is toxic in large amounts. Selenium protects intracellular structures against oxidative damage. It is an essential component of glutathione peroxidase. [NIH]

Serum: The clear portion of any body fluid; the clear fluid moistening serous membranes. 2. blood serum; the clear liquid that separates from blood on clotting. 3. immune serum; blood serum from an immunized animal used for passive immunization; an antiserum; antitoxin, or antivenin. [EU]

Somatic: 1. pertaining to or characteristic of the soma or body. 2. pertaining to the body wall in contrast to the viscera. [EU]

Species: A taxonomic category subordinate to a genus (or subgenus) and superior to a subspecies or variety, composed of individuals possessing common characters distinguishing them from other categories of individuals of the same taxonomic level. In taxonomic nomenclature, species are designated by the genus name followed by a Latin or Latinized adjective or noun. [EU]

Substrate: A substance upon which an enzyme acts. [EU]

Tyrosine: A non-essential amino acid. In animals it is synthesized from phenylalanine. It is also the precursor of epinephrine, thyroid hormones, and melanin. [NIH]

CHAPTER 4. PATENTS ON POLYCYSTIC KIDNEY DISEASE

Overview

You can learn about innovations relating to polycystic kidney disease by reading recent patents and patent applications. Patents can be physical innovations (e.g. chemicals, pharmaceuticals, medical equipment) or processes (e.g. treatments or diagnostic procedures). The United States Patent and Trademark Office defines a patent as a grant of a property right to the inventor, issued by the Patent and Trademark Office.[21] Patents, therefore, are intellectual property. For the United States, the term of a new patent is 20 years from the date when the patent application was filed. If the inventor wishes to receive economic benefits, it is likely that the invention will become commercially available to patients with polycystic kidney disease within 20 years of the initial filing. It is important to understand, therefore, that an inventor's patent does not indicate that a product or service is or will be commercially available to patients with polycystic kidney disease. The patent implies only that the inventor has "the right to exclude others from making, using, offering for sale, or selling" the invention in the United States. While this relates to U.S. patents, similar rules govern foreign patents.

In this chapter, we show you how to locate information on patents and their inventors. If you find a patent that is particularly interesting to you, contact the inventor or the assignee for further information.

[21] Adapted from The U. S. Patent and Trademark Office:
http://www.uspto.gov/web/offices/pac/doc/general/whatis.htm.

Patents on Polycystic Kidney Disease

By performing a patent search focusing on polycystic kidney disease, you can obtain information such as the title of the invention, the names of the inventor(s), the assignee(s) or the company that owns or controls the patent, a short abstract that summarizes the patent, and a few excerpts from the description of the patent. The abstract of a patent tends to be more technical in nature, while the description is often written for the public. Full patent descriptions contain much more information than is presented here (e.g. claims, references, figures, diagrams, etc.). We will tell you how to obtain this information later in the chapter. The following is an example of the type of information that you can expect to obtain from a patent search on polycystic kidney disease:

- **Polycystic kidney disease 1 gene and uses thereof**

  Inventor(s): Harris; Peter Charles (Oxford, GB), Peral; Belen (Oxford, GB), Ward; Christopher J. (Oxford, GB), Hughes; James (Oxford, GB), Breuning; Martin Hendrik (Zaandam, NL), Peters; Dorothea Johanna Maria (Leiden, NL), Roelfsema; Jeroen Hendrik (Leiden, NL), Sampson; Julian (Cardiff, GB), Halley; Dirkje Jorijntje Johanna (Rotterdam, NL), Nellist; Mark David (Rotterdam, NL), Janssen; Lambertus Antonius Jacobus (Barendrecht, NL), Hesseling; Ajenne Lique Wilhelma (Spijkenisse, NL)

  Assignee(s): Medical Research Council (GB)

  Patent Number: 6,380,360

  Date filed: March 31, 1998

  Abstract: The present invention relates to the polycystic kidney disease 1 (PKD1) gene and its nucleic acid sequence, mutations thereof in patients having PKD1-associated disorders, the protein encoded by the PKD1 gene or its mutants, and their uses in disease diagnosis and therapy.

  Excerpt(s): In humans, one of the commonest of all genetic disorders is autosomal dominant polycystic kidney disease (ADPKD) also termed adult polycystic kidney disease (APKD), affecting approximately 1/1000 individuals (Dalgaard, 1957). ADPKD is a progressive disease of cyst formation and enlargement typically leading to end stage renal disease (ESRD) in late middle age. The major cause of morbidity in ADPKD is progressive renal disease characterized by the formation and enlargement of fluid filled cysts, resulting in grossly enlarged kidneys. Renal function deteriorates as normal tissue is compromised by cystic growth, resulting in end stage renal disease (ESRD) in more than 50% of patients by the age of 60 years (Gabow, et al., 1992). ADPKD accounts for

8-10% of all renal transplantation and dialysis patients in Europe and the USA (Gabow, 1993). ... The first step towards positional cloning of an ADPKD gene was the demonstration of linkage of one locus now designated the polycystic kidney disease 1 (PKD1) locus to the .alpha. globin cluster on the short arm of chromosome 16 (Reeders, et al., 1985). Subsequently, families with ADPKD unlinked to markers on 16p were described (Kimberling, et al., 1988; Romeo, et al., 1988) and a second ADPKD locus (PKD2) has recently been assigned to chromosome region 4q13-q23 (Kimberling, et al., 1993; Peter, et al., 1993). It is estimated that approximately 85% of ADPKD is due to PKD1 (Peters and Sankuijl, 1992) with PKD2 accounting for most of the remainder. PKD2 appears to be milder condition with a later age of onset and ESRD (Parfrey, et al., 1990; Gabow, et al., 1992; Ravine, et al., 1992). ... Disease associated genomic rearrangements, detected by cytogenetics or pulsed field gel electrophoresis (PFGE) have been instrumental in the identification of various genes associated with various genetic disorders. Hitherto, no such abnormalities related to PKD1 have been described. This situation contrasts with that for the tuberous sclerosis locus, which lies within 16p13.3 (TSC2) In that case, TSC associated deletions were detected by PFGE within the interval thought to contain the PKD1 gene and their characterisation was a significant step toward the rapid identification of the TSC2 gene (European Chromosome 16 Tuberous Sclerosis Consortium, 1993). The TSC2 gene therefore maps within the candidate region for the hitherto unidentified PKD1 gene; as polycystic kidneys are a feature common to TSC and ADPKD1 (Bernstein and Robbins, 1991) the possibility of an etiological link, as proposed by Kandt et al. (1992), was considered. A contiguous gene syndrome resulting from the disruption of PKD1 and the adjacent tuberous sclerosis 2 (TSC2) gene, which is associated with TSC and severe childhood onset polycystic kidney disease, has also been defined (Brook-Carter et al., 1994).

Web site: http://www.delphion.com/details?pn=US06380360__

- **Identification of polycystic kidney disease gene, diagnostics and treatment**

  Inventor(s): Reeders; Stephen (Newtonville, MA), Schneider; Michael (Boston, MA), Glucksmann; Maria Alexandra (Somerville, MA)

  Assignee(s): Brigham and Women's Hospital (Boston, MA), Millenium Pharmaceuticals (Cambridge, MA)

  Patent Number: 5,891,628

  Date filed: June 2, 1995

Abstract: The present invention relates to the identification of the autosomal dominant polycystic kidney disease (PKD) gene and high throughput assays to identify compounds that interfere with PKD activity. Interfering compounds that inhibit the expression, synthesis and/or bioactivity of the PKD gene product can be used therapeutically to treat polycystic kidney disease.

Excerpt(s): The present invention relates to the identification of the gene, referred to as the PKD1 gene, mutations in which are responsible for the vast majority of cases involving autosomal dominant polycystic kidney disease (ADPKD). The PKD1 gene, including the complete nucleotide sequence of the gene's coding region are presented. Further, the complete PKD1 gene product amino acid sequence and protein structure and antibodies directed against the PKD1 gene product are also presented. Additionally, the present invention relates to therapeutic methods and compositions for the treatment of ADPKD symptoms. Methods are also presented for the identification of compounds that modulate the level of expression of the PKD1 gene or the activity of mutant PKD1 gene product, and the evaluation and use of such compounds in the treatment of ADPKD symptoms. Still further, the present invention relates to prognostic and diagnostic, including prenatal, methods and compositions for the detection of mutant PKD1 alleles and/or abnormal levels of PKD1 gene product or gene product activity. ... Autosomal dominant polycystic kidney disease (ADPKD) is among the most prevalent dominant human disorders, affecting between 1 in 1,000 and 1 in 3,000 individuals worldwide (Dalgaard, O. Z., 1957, Acta. Med. Scand. 158:1-251). The major manifestation of the disorder is the progressive cystic dilation of renal tubules (Gabow, P. A., 1990, Am. J. Kidney Dis. 16:403-413), leading to renal failure in half of affected individuals by age 50. ... The present invention relates to methods and compositions for the diagnosis and treatment of autosomal dominant polycystic kidney disease (ADPKD). Specifically, a novel gene, referred to as the PKD1 gene, is described in Section 5.1. Mutations within the PKD1 gene are responsible for approximately 90% cases of ADPKD. Additionally, the PKD1 gene product, including the nucleotide sequence of the complete coding region is described in Section 5.2. Antibodies directed against the PKD1 gene product are described in Section 5.3.

Web site: http://www.delphion.com/details?pn=US05891628__

Patent Applications on Polycystic Kidney Disease

As of December 2000, U.S. patent applications are open to public viewing.[22] Applications are patent requests which have yet to be granted (the process to achieve a patent can take several years). The following patent applications have been filed since December 2000 relating to polycystic kidney disease:

- **Polycystic kidney disease PKD2 gene and uses thereof**

  Inventor(s): Somlo, Stefan ; (Westport, CT), Mochizuki, Toshio ; (Tokyo, JP)

  Correspondence: Amster, Rothstein & Ebenstein; Attorneys for Applicants; 90 Park Avenue; New York; NY; 10016; US

  Patent Application Number: 20020061520

  Date filed: January 2, 2001

  Abstract: The present invention provides a purified and isolated wild type PKD2 gene, as well as mutated forms of this gene. The present invention also provides one or more single-stranded nucleic acid probes which specifically hybridize to the wild type PKD2 gene or the mutated PKD2 gene, and mixtures thereof, which may be formulated in kits, and used in the diagnosis of ADPKD associated with the mutated PKD2 gene. The present invention also provides a method for diagnosing ADPKD caused by a mutated PKD2 gene, as well as a method for treating autosomal dominant polycystic kidney disease caused by a mutated PKD2 gene.

  Excerpt(s): This invention is based upon the discovery by the inventors of the PKD2 gene associated with Autosomal Dominant Polycystic Kidney Disease ("ADPKD"), the "PKD2 gene" or "PKD2", and a novel protein encoded by this gene. The discovery of the PKD2 gene and the protein encoded by the gene will have important implications in the diagnosis and treatment of ADPKD caused by defects in the PKD2 gene. ... ADPKD is a genetically heterogeneous disorder that affects approximately 500,000 Americans and five million individuals world wide, and accounts for 8 to 10% of all end stage renal disease (ESRD) worldwide (Gabow, P. A. N. Eng. J. Med. 329:332 (1993)). Its principal clinical manifestation is bilateral renal cysts that result in chronic renal failure in about 45% of affected individuals by age 60 (Gabow, P. A., supra). Hypertension and liver cysts are common, and the involvement of other organ systems (Gabow, P. A., et al. Kidney Int. 38:1177 (1990); Chapman, A. B., et al. N. Eng. J. Med. 327:916 (1992); Hossack, K. F., et al. N. Enc. J. Med. 319:907 (1988); Torres,

---

[22] This has been a common practice outside the United States prior to December 2000.

V. E., et al. Am. J. Kidney Dis. 22:513 (1993); Huston, J., et al. J. Am. Soc. Nephrol. 3:1871 (1993); Somlo, S., et al. J. Am. Soc. NeDhrol. 4:1371 (1993)) lends support to the view that polycystic kidney disease is a systemic disorder (Gabow, P. A., supra). ... To date, most forms of ADPKD have been associated with two genes, PKD1 and PKD2. The full genomic structure and cDNA sequence for the PKD1 gene has been identified (The International Polycystic Kidney Disease Consortium, Cell 81:289 (1995); The American PKD1 Consortium, Hum. Mol. Genet. 4:575 (1995)). Mutations in the PKD1 gene are suspected of causing 80-90% of all cases of ADPKD. The PKD2 gene has been localized on chromosome 4q21-23 and accounts for approximately 15% of affected families (Kimberling, W. J., et al. Genomics 18:467 (1993); Peters, D. J. M. and L. A. Sandkuijl Contrib. Neohrol. 97:128 (1992)). Prior to the present invention, however, the PKD2 gene had not been identified.

Web site: http://appft1.uspto.gov/netahtml/PTO/search-bool.html

Keeping Current

In order to stay informed about patents and patent applications dealing with polycystic kidney disease, you can access the U.S. Patent Office archive via the Internet at no cost to you. This archive is available at the following Web address: **http://www.uspto.gov/main/patents.htm**. Under "Services," click on "Search Patents." You will see two broad options: (1) Patent Grants, and (2) Patent Applications. To see a list of granted patents, perform the following steps: Under "Patent Grants," click "Quick Search." Then, type "polycystic kidney disease" (or synonyms) into the "Term 1" box. After clicking on the search button, scroll down to see the various patents which have been granted to date on polycystic kidney disease. You can also use this procedure to view pending patent applications concerning polycystic kidney disease. Simply go back to the following Web address: **http://www.uspto.gov/main/patents.htm**. Under "Services," click on "Search Patents." Select "Quick Search" under "Patent Applications." Then proceed with the steps listed above.

CHAPTER 5. BOOKS ON POLYCYSTIC KIDNEY DISEASE

Overview

This chapter provides bibliographic book references relating to polycystic kidney disease. You have many options to locate books on polycystic kidney disease. The simplest method is to go to your local bookseller and inquire about titles that they have in stock or can special order for you. Some patients, however, feel uncomfortable approaching their local booksellers and prefer online sources (e.g. **www.amazon.com** and **www.bn.com**). In addition to online booksellers, excellent sources for book titles on polycystic kidney disease include the Combined Health Information Database and the National Library of Medicine. Once you have found a title that interests you, visit your local public or medical library to see if it is available for loan.

Book Summaries: Federal Agencies

The Combined Health Information Database collects various book abstracts from a variety of healthcare institutions and federal agencies. To access these summaries, go to **http://chid.nih.gov/detail/detail.html**. You will need to use the "Detailed Search" option. To find book summaries, use the drop boxes at the bottom of the search page where "You may refine your search by." Select the dates and language you prefer. For the format option, select "Monograph/Book." Now type "polycystic kidney disease" (or synonyms) into the "For these words:" box. You will only receive results on books. You should check back periodically with this database which is updated every 3 months. The following is a typical result when searching for books on polycystic kidney disease:

- **Proceedings of the Fifth International Workshop on Polycystic Kidney Disease**

Source: Kansas City, MO: PKR Foundation. 1993. 181 p.

Contact: Available from PKR Foundation. 4901 Main Street, Suite 320, Kansas City, MO 64112. (800) 753-2873. Price: $33.95 for members; $39 for nonmembers. ISBN: 096145671X.

Summary: The articles gathered in this book are the result of presentations of papers on research at the 5th International Workshop on Polycystic Kidney Disease, held in Kansas City, Missouri in June 1992. Twenty-two brief chapters are presented in four sections: the genetics of polycystic kidney disease (PKD); the clinical aspects of autosomal dominant PKD; acquired renal cystic disease; and the cell biology of PKD. These chapters include brief reference lists. The remainder of the book consists of 41 abstracts accepted for poster presentation at the conference.

- **PKD Patient's Manual: Understanding and Living with Autosomal Dominant Polycystic Kidney Disease. 2nd ed**

Source: Kansas City, MO: Polycystic Kidney Research Foundation (PKR Foundation). 1995. 66 p.

Contact: Available from Polycystic Kidney Research Foundation (PKR Foundation). 4901 Main Street, Suite 320, Kansas City, MO 64112-2674. (800) 753-2873 or (816) 931-2600. Price: $10.00 (members); $15.00 (nonmembers), as of 1996. ISBN: 0961456744.

Summary: This book provides information about autosomal dominant polycystic kidney disease (ADPKD) to those who have the disease, those who are at risk due to an affected parent, and interested family members and friends. Topics include the nature of the disease and its prevalence, how ADPKD is inherited, diagnostic tests, basic kidney anatomy and physiology, kidney cysts and how they form, signs and symptoms of ADPKD, the role of dialysis or transplantation in the treatment, pregnancy in women with ADPKD, preventive diet therapy, managing children with ADPKD, symptoms of kidney failure, and the role of self care. The book is written primarily in question and answer format, with most medical terms avoided or explained in layperson's language. 12 figures. 1 table. 5 references.

Book Summaries: Online Booksellers

Commercial Internet-based booksellers, such as Amazon.com and Barnes & Noble.com, offer summaries which have been supplied by each title's publisher. Some summaries also include customer reviews. Your local bookseller may have access to in-house and commercial databases that index all published books (e.g. Books in Print®). The following have been recently listed with online booksellers as relating to polycystic kidney disease (sorted alphabetically by title; follow the hyperlink to view more details at Amazon.com):

- **Autosomal Dominant Polycystic Kidney Desease: Seminar on Autosomal Dominant Polycystic Kidney Disease, Vimercate, June 18, 1994 (Contributions to nep** by Seminar on Autosomal Dominant Polycystic Kidney Disease (1995); ISBN: 3805560907; http://www.amazon.com/exec/obidos/ASIN/3805560907/icongroupin terna

- **Cystic Kidney (Developments in Nephrology, No 27)** by Kenneth D. Gardner, Jay Bernstein (Editor) (1990); ISBN: 079230392X; http://www.amazon.com/exec/obidos/ASIN/079230392X/icongroupi nterna

- **Polycystic Kidney Disease (Contributions to Nephrology, Vol 97)** by M.H. Breuning, et al (1992); ISBN: 3805555865; http://www.amazon.com/exec/obidos/ASIN/3805555865/icongroupin terna

- **Polycystic Kidney Disease (Oxford Clinical Nephrology Series)** by Michael L. Watson (Editor), et al; ISBN: 0192625780; http://www.amazon.com/exec/obidos/ASIN/0192625780/icongroupin terna

- **Problems in diagnosis and management of polycystic kidney disease : proceedings of the First International Workshop on Polycystic Kidney Disease** ; ISBN: 0961456701; http://www.amazon.com/exec/obidos/ASIN/0961456701/icongroupin terna

The National Library of Medicine Book Index

The National Library of Medicine at the National Institutes of Health has a massive database of books published on healthcare and biomedicine. Go to the following Internet site, **http://locatorplus.gov/**, and then select "Search LOCATORplus." Once you are in the search area, simply type "polycystic kidney disease" (or synonyms) into the search box, and select "books only." From there, results can be sorted by publication date, author, or relevance. The following was recently catalogued by the National Library of Medicine.[23]

- **Adult polycystic kidney diseases.**   Author: Manuel Martínez-Maldonado; Year: 1976; Oklahoma City: National Kidney Foundation, 1976

- **Autosomal dominant polycystic kidney disease.**   Author: volume editors, A. Sessa ... [et al.]; Year: 1995; Basel; New York: Karger, 1995; ISBN: 3805560907 (hardcover)
  http://www.amazon.com/exec/obidos/ASIN/3805560907/icongroupinterna

- **Bilateral polycystic disease of the kidneys; a follow-up of two hundred and eighty-four patients and their families. [Tr. from the Danish].** Author: Dalgaard, O. Z; Year: 1957; Copenhagen, Munksgaard, 1957

- **Cystic diseases of the kidney.**   Author: William L. Henrich; Year: 1994; [Dallas, Tex.]: University of Texas Southwestern Medical Center, 1994

- **Hypertension and vascular studies in congenital polycystic kidney.** Author: Schacht, Frederick William, 1898-; Year: 1930; [Minneapolis] 1930

- **Kidney disease in primary care.**   Author: editors, Anil K. Mandal, N. Stanley Nahman, Jr; Year: 1998; Baltimore, MD: Williams & Wilkins, c1998; ISBN: 0683300571
  http://www.amazon.com/exec/obidos/ASIN/0683300571/icongroupinterna

- **Kidney disease quality of life short form (KDQOL-SF), version 1.3: a manual for use and scoring.** Author: Ron D. Hays ... [et al.]; Year: 1997; Santa Monica, CA: Rand, 1997

- **Kidney disease quality of life short form (KDQOL-SFtm), version 1.2: a manual for use and scoring.**   Author: Ron D. Hays; Year: 1995; Santa Monica, CA: Rand, 1996

- **Multicystic dysplastic kidney: a clinical and pathological study of 29 cases.** Author: Feinzaig, Willy, 1931-; Year: 1964; [Minneapolis] 1964

---

[23] In addition to LOCATORPlus, in collaboration with authors and publishers, the National Center for Biotechnology Information (NCBI) is adapting biomedical books for the Web. The books may be accessed in two ways: (1) by searching directly using any search term or phrase (in the same way as the bibliographic database PubMed), or (2) by following the links to PubMed abstracts. Each PubMed abstract has a "Books" button that displays a facsimile of the abstract in which some phrases are hypertext links. These phrases are also found in the books available at NCBI. Click on hyperlinked results in the list of books in which the phrase is found. Currently, the majority of the links are between the books and PubMed. In the future, more links will be created between the books and other types of information, such as gene and protein sequences and macromolecular structures. See **http://www.ncbi.nlm.nih.gov/entrez/query.fcgi?db=Books.**

- **Polycystic kidney disease: hereditary and acquired.** Author: Jared J. Grantham; Year: 1984; New York, NY (2 Park Ave, New York 10016): National Kidney Foundation, c1984

- **Polycystic kidney disease in children.** Author: Uhler, Walter Miller, 1918-; Year: 1951; [Minneapolis] 1951

- **Polycystic kidney disease.** Author: edited by Michael L. Watson and Vicente E. Torres; Year: 1996; Oxford; New York: Oxford University Press, 1996; ISBN: 0192625780 (hbk)
  http://www.amazon.com/exec/obidos/ASIN/0192625780/icongroupin terna

- **Polycystic kidney disease.** Author: 2nd Int. Workshop of the European Concerted Action Towards Prevention of Renal Failure Caused by Polycystic Kidney Disease, Parma, September 20/21, 1991; volume editors, M.H. Breuning, M. Devoto, G. Romeo; Year: 1992; Basel; New York: Karger, 1992; ISBN: 3805555865 (alk. paper)
  http://www.amazon.com/exec/obidos/ASIN/3805555865/icongroupin terna

- **Problems in diagnosis and management of polycystic kidney disease: proceedings of the First International Workshop on Polycystic Kidney Disease.** Author: Jared J. Grantham, Kenneth D. Gardner, editors; Year: 1985; Kansas City [Mo.]: PKR Foundation, c1985; ISBN: 0961456701
  http://www.amazon.com/exec/obidos/ASIN/0961456701/icongroupin terna

- **Psychosocial effects of genetic testing in adult polycystic kidney disease: final report.** Author: Ellen Rosenberg ... [et al.]; Year: 1991; [Québec]: Conseil québécois de la recherche sociale, [1991]

Chapters on Polycystic Kidney Disease

Frequently, polycystic kidney disease will be discussed within a book, perhaps within a specific chapter. In order to find chapters that are specifically dealing with polycystic kidney disease, an excellent source of abstracts is the Combined Health Information Database. You will need to limit your search to book chapters and polycystic kidney disease using the "Detailed Search" option. Go directly to the following hyperlink: **http://chid.nih.gov/detail/detail.html**. To find book chapters, use the drop boxes at the bottom of the search page where "You may refine your search by." Select the dates and language you prefer, and the format option "Book Chapter." By making these selections and typing in "polycystic kidney disease" (or synonyms) into the "For these words:" box, you will only receive results on chapters in books. The following is a typical result when searching for book chapters on polycystic kidney disease:

- **Polycystic Kidney Disease: Hereditary and Acquired**

  Source: in Stollerman, G.H., et al., eds. Advances in Internal Medicine. Vol 38. St. Louis, MO: Mosby-Year Book, Inc. 1993. p. 409-420.

  Contact: Available from Mosby Year-Book, Inc. 11830 Westline Industrial Drive, St. Louis, MO 63146. (800) 426-4545. Fax (800) 535-9935. E-mail: customer.support@mosby.com. Price: $72.95. ISBN: 0815183089. ISSN:00652822.

  Summary: This chapter reviews hereditary and acquired polycystic kidney disease (PKD). The author addresses recent advances in understanding the etiology and pathogenesis of cysts and in the clinical management of the major clinical forms of renal cystic disease. It is now established that in 90 percent of cases, the autosomal dominant form of PKD is the result of a mutation on chromosome 16. The condition typically causes renal failure in the fifth and sixth decades of life, but cysts can be identified early in childhood and even in utero. The clinician should be aware that members of families with hereditary PKD may present with symptomatic cysts in numerous other organs, including the liver, which is affected in approximately 50 percent of the cases, the spleen, pancreas, and pineal gland. More ominously, hereditary PKD is associated with an increased incidence of cerebral artery aneurisms and mitral and aortic valve involvement. Acquired PKD is being recognized increasingly as the result of prolonged maintenance of dialysis patients with end-stage renal disease (ESRD). Bilateral cysts develop in the failing kidney, at times early in the course of renal failure. Their formation now is established to be the direct result of the uremic state, and cyst formation can be stopped and reversed with correction of uremia by, for example, renal transplantation. More seriously, a significant number of such acquired renal cysts undergo malignant change with occasional distant metastases. One of the questions now under consideration is whether nephrectomy, with its risks, should be considered in patients with acquired PKD with the aim of preventing the consequences of renal malignancy. 81 references. (AA-M).

- **Autosomal Recessive Polycystic Kidney Disease**

  Source: in Gardner, K.D.; Bernstein, J., eds. The Cystic Kidney. Hingham, MA: Kluwer Academic Publishers. 1990. p. 327-350.

Contact: Available from Kluwer Academic Publishers. P.O. Box 358, Accord Station, Hingham, MA 02018. (617) 871-6600. Price: $184.50 (as of 1994). ISBN: 079230392X. Orders must be prepaid.

Summary: Autosomal recessive polycystic kidney disease (ARPKD) is a specific disease of the kidneys and liver, characterized by renal collecting tubule ectasia and invariably accompanied by biliary dysgenesis and portal fibrosis. This chapter, from a book about renal cysts and cystic kidneys, describes the evolution of knowledge about ARPKD, the diagnosis and management of the condition, and a summary of what is known about pathogenetic mechanisms. Topics include a historical perspective, comparison of ARKPD with other renal cystic diseases, clinical manifestations, radiologic assessment, gross and microscopic pathology, genetics, patient survival, and diagnosis and management of the condition. 7 figures. 5 tables. 66 references.

- **Natural History of Autosomal Dominant Polycystic Kidney Disease**

Source: in Coggins, C.H.; Hancock, E.W., Eds. Annual Review of Medicine: Selected Topics in the Clinical Sciences, Volume 45. Palo Alto, CA: Annual Reviews Inc. 1994. p. 23-29.

Contact: Available from Annual Reviews Inc. 4139 El Camino Way, P.O. Box 10139, Palo Alto, CA 94303-0139. (800) 523-8635. Fax: (415) 855-9815. Price: $47. ISBN: 0824305450.

Summary: This chapter, from an Annual Review of Medicine, discusses the natural history of autosomal dominant polycystic kidney disease (PKD). The authors note that at least two different genes, which have been mapped to chromosomes 4 and 16, cause autosomal dominant PKD, a disorder with renal and extrarenal manifestations. The renal disease is characterized clinically by hypertension, acute and chronic pain, and variable progression to end-stage renal disease. Extrarenal manifestations include liver cysts, which may lead to complications; ruptured intracranial aneurysms; cardiac valvular disease; colonic diverticula; and inguinal hernias. 1 table. 28 references. (AA-M).

- **Inherited Kidney Diseases: Polycystic Kidney Disease and Alport Syndrome**

Source: in Schrier, R.W., et al., eds. Advances in Internal Medicine. Vol 40. St. Louis, MO: Mosby-Year Book, Inc. 1995. p. 303-339.

Contact: Available from Mosby Year-Book, Inc. 11830 Westline Industrial Drive, St. Louis, MO 63146. (800) 426-4545. Fax (800) 535-9935. E-mail: customer.support@mosby.com. Price: $72.95. ISBN: 0815183135. ISSN: 00652822.

Summary: Recent advances in DNA technology have led to explosive growth in the knowledge of the molecular genetics in many inherited disorders, including kidney diseases. This progress has improved the understanding of pathogenesis, has modified the classification of these diseases, and has changed clinical attitudes. Along with these advances, new ethical issues concerning prenatal diagnosis and presymptomatic testing have been raised, most particularly in late-onset inherited disorders. All these issues are exemplified in polycystic kidney disease (PKD) and in Alport syndrome, which are the most prevalent hereditary kidney diseases in adults and the basis of this review chapter. The first section covers autosomal dominant polycystic kidney disease (ADPKD), including its genetics and epidemiology, renal manifestations, hypertension, renal failure and its progression, patient care management, extrarenal manifestations (liver involvement, intracranial aneurysms, cardiovascular changes), and diagnosis and genetic counseling. The second section addresses Alport syndrome, an inherited disorder characterized by progressive nephritis with hematuria and sensorineural hearing loss. Topics in this section include clinical findings, pathology and pathogenesis, molecular genetics, and treatment specifics. Regular dialysis and kidney transplantation are common means of treatment of patients with Alport syndrome when end-stage renal disease (ESRD) has been reached. 4 figures. 3 tables. 115 references.

- **Autosomal Dominant Polycystic Kidney Disease**

Source: in Gardner, K.D.; Berstein, J., eds. The Cystic Kidney. Hingham, MA: Kluwer Academic Publishers. 1990. p. 296-326.

Contact: Available from Kluwer Academic Publishers. P.O. Box 358, Accord Station, Hingham, MA 02018. (617) 871-6600. Price: $184.50 (as of 1994). ISBN: 079230392X. Orders must be prepaid.

Summary: This chapter, from a book about renal cysts and cystic kidneys, discusses autosomal dominant polycystic kidney disease (ADPKD). The author provides a definition of the condition; its pathogenesis; the role of inheritance; epidemiology; methods of diagnosis, including clinical, routine laboratory studies, radiographic studies, and gene linkage analysis; and clinical manifestations, including symptoms and signs, laboratory data, renal pathology, renal infection, nephrolithiasis and intrarenal calcification, and renal malignancy. The author also discusses extrarenal manifestations of ADPKD, including gastrointestinal manifestations, cardiac manifestations, and vascular manifestations; and the natural history and treatment of ADPKD. 3 figures. 9 tables. 185 references.

Directories

In addition to the references and resources discussed earlier in this chapter, a number of directories relating to polycystic kidney disease have been published that consolidate information across various sources. These too might be useful in gaining access to additional guidance on polycystic kidney disease. The Combined Health Information Database lists the following, which you may wish to consult in your local medical library:[24]

- **1998-1999 Complete Directory for People with Rare Disorders**

  Source: Lakeville, CT: Grey House Publishing, Inc. 1998. 726 p.

  Contact: Available from Grey House Publishing, Inc. Pocket Knife Square, Lakeville, CT 06039. (860) 435-0868. Fax (860) 435-0867. Price: $190.00. ISBN: 0939300982.

  Summary: This directory from the National Organization for Rare Disorders (NORD) provides a wealth of information on diseases and organizations. The directory offers four sections: disease descriptions, disease specific organizations, umbrella organizations, and Government agencies. In the first section, the directory includes descriptions of 1,102 rare diseases in alphabetical order. Each entry defines the disorder, then refers readers to organizations that might be of interest. Diseases related to kidney and urologic diseases are Alport syndrome, Bartter's syndrome, blue diaper syndrome, branchiotorenal syndrome, renal cell carcinoma, citrullinemia, cystinuria, Drash syndrome, Fraser syndrome, Galloway Mowat syndrome, Golderhar syndrome, Goodpasture syndrome, benign familial hematuria, hemolytic uremic syndrome, hepatic fibrosis, IgA nephropathy, interstitial cystitis, Loken senior syndrome, medullary cystic disease, medullary sponge kidney, Mullerian aplasia, multiple myeloma, nail patella syndrome, Ochoa syndrome, Peyronie disease, polycystic kidney diseases, prostatitis, purpura, renal agenesis, renal glycosuria, WAGR syndrome, Wegener's granulomatosis, and Wilms tumor. Each of the 445 organizations listed in the second section is associated with a specific disease or group of diseases. In addition to contact information, there is a descriptive paragraph about the

---

[24] You will need to limit your search to "Directories" and polycystic kidney disease using the "Detailed Search" option. Go directly to the following hyperlink: **http://chid.nih.gov/detail/detail.html**. To find directories, use the drop boxes at the bottom of the search page where "You may refine your search by". For publication date, select "All Years", select language and the format option "Directory". By making these selections and typing in "polycystic kidney disease" (or synonyms) into the "For these words:" box, you will only receive results on directories dealing with polycystic kidney disease. You should check back periodically with this database as it is updated every three months.

organization and its primary goals and program activities. Entries include materials published by the organization as well as the diseases the organization covers. The third section lists 444 organizations that are more general in nature, serving a wide range of diseases (for example, the American Liver Foundation). The final section describes 74 agencies that are important Federal Government contacts that serve the diverse needs of individuals with rare disorders. A name and keyword index concludes the volume.

- **Research Program 1995-1996**

  Source: New York, NY: National Kidney Foundation. 1995. 68 p.

  Contact: Available from National Kidney Foundation. 30 East 33rd Street, New York, NY 10016. (800) 622-9010. Price: Single copy free.

  Summary: This Research Program book lists the recipients of the National Kidney Foundation's various fellowships and grants and summarizes their projects for 1995-1996. The foundation provides four channels for research funding: Research Fellowships, Young Investigator Grants, the Clinical Scientist Award, and Affiliate Research Awards. The book provides the name of the researcher, his or her affiliation, an abstract of the work being undertaken, and a summary of the researcher's vitae. Funded research includes work in the areas of polycystic kidney disease; glomerular filtration; animal studies; genetics; diabetic kidney disease; sodium metabolism; hypertension; the nephrotic syndrome; renal allograft rejection; HIV-associated nephropathy; glomerulonephritis; and cystinuria.

General Home References

In addition to references for polycystic kidney disease, you may want a general home medical guide that spans all aspects of home healthcare. The following list is a recent sample of such guides (sorted alphabetically by title; hyperlinks provide rankings, information, and reviews at Amazon.com):

- **Urodynamics Made Easy** by Christopher R. Chapple, Scott A. MacDiarmid; Paperback -- 2nd edition (April 15, 2000), Churchill Livingstone; ISBN: 0443054630;
  http://www.amazon.com/exec/obidos/ASIN/0443054630/icongroupinterna

Vocabulary Builder

Androgens: A class of sex hormones associated with the development and maintenance of the secondary male sex characteristics, sperm induction, and sexual differentiation. In addition to increasing virility and libido, they also increase nitrogen and water retention and stimulate skeletal growth. [NIH]

Aplasia: Lack of development of an organ or tissue, or of the cellular products from an organ or tissue. [EU]

Calcification: The process by which organic tissue becomes hardened by a deposit of calcium salts within its substance. [EU]

Cardiovascular: Pertaining to the heart and blood vessels. [EU]

Cystinuria: An inherited abnormality of renal tubular transport of dibasic amino acids leading to massive urinary excretion of cystine, lysine, arginine, and ornithine. [NIH]

Cystitis: Inflammation of the urinary bladder. [EU]

Dementia: An acquired organic mental disorder with loss of intellectual abilities of sufficient severity to interfere with social or occupational functioning. The dysfunction is multifaceted and involves memory, behavior, personality, judgment, attention, spatial relations, language, abstract thought, and other executive functions. The intellectual decline is usually progressive, and initially spares the level of consciousness. [NIH]

Dysgenesis: Defective development. [EU]

Glycosuria: The presence of glucose in the urine; especially the excretion of an abnormally large amount of sugar (glucose) in the urine, i.e., more than 1 gm. in 24 hours. [EU]

Hernia: The protrusion of a loop or knuckle of an organ or tissue through an abnormal opening. [EU]

Insulin: A protein hormone secreted by beta cells of the pancreas. Insulin plays a major role in the regulation of glucose metabolism, generally promoting the cellular utilization of glucose. It is also an important regulator of protein and lipid metabolism. Insulin is used as a drug to control insulin-dependent diabetes mellitus. [NIH]

Interstitial: Pertaining to or situated between parts or in the interspaces of a tissue. [EU]

Malignant: Tending to become progressively worse and to result in death. Having the properties of anaplasia, invasion, and metastasis; said of tumours. [EU]

Myeloma: A tumour composed of cells of the type normally found in the bone marrow. [EU]

Nephropathy: Disease of the kidneys. [EU]

Nephrotic: Pertaining to, resembling, or caused by nephrosis. [EU]

Ovary: Either of the paired glands in the female that produce the female germ cells and secrete some of the female sex hormones. [NIH]

Pancreatitis: Acute or chronic inflammation of the pancreas, which may be asymptomatic or symptomatic, and which is due to autodigestion of a pancreatic tissue by its own enzymes. It is caused most often by alcoholism or biliary tract disease; less commonly it may be associated with hyperlipaemia, hyperparathyroidism, abdominal trauma (accidental or operative injury), vasculitis, or uraemia. [EU]

Patella: The flat, triangular bone situated at the anterior part of the knee. [NIH]

Prevalence: The total number of cases of a given disease in a specified population at a designated time. It is differentiated from incidence, which refers to the number of new cases in the population at a given time. [NIH]

Purpura: Purplish or brownish red discoloration, easily visible through the epidermis, caused by hemorrhage into the tissues. [NIH]

CHAPTER 6. MULTIMEDIA ON POLYCYSTIC KIDNEY DISEASE

Overview

Information on polycystic kidney disease can come in a variety of formats. Among multimedia sources, video productions, slides, audiotapes, and computer databases are often available. In this chapter, we show you how to keep current on multimedia sources of information on polycystic kidney disease. We start with sources that have been summarized by federal agencies, and then show you how to find bibliographic information catalogued by the National Library of Medicine. If you see an interesting item, visit your local medical library to check on the availability of the title.

Video Recordings

Most diseases do not have a video dedicated to them. If they do, they are often rather technical in nature. An excellent source of multimedia information on polycystic kidney disease is the Combined Health Information Database. You will need to limit your search to "video recording" and "polycystic kidney disease" using the "Detailed Search" option. Go to the following hyperlink: **http://chid.nih.gov/detail/detail.html**. To find video productions, use the drop boxes at the bottom of the search page where "You may refine your search by." Select the dates and language you prefer, and the format option "Videorecording (videotape, videocassette, etc.)." By making these selections and typing "polycystic kidney disease" (or synonyms) into the "For these words:" box, you will only receive results on video productions. The following is a typical result when searching for video recordings on polycystic kidney disease:

- **Choices: Options for Living with Kidney Failure**

  Source: McGaw Park, IL: Baxter Healthcare Corporation. 1997 (videocassette).

  Contact: Available from community service section of Blockbuster video stores. Price: Free rental. Also available to health professionals from Baxter Healthcare Corporation. (888) 736-2543. 1620 Waukegan Road, McGaw Park, IL 60085.

  Summary: This videotape program helps viewers newly diagnosed with kidney failure to understand their treatment options and to make more informed choices for their own health care. The narrator reminds viewers that many members make up the health care team, but stresses that patients are the most important member of that team. The program reviews the functions of the kidneys, including clean the blood, make red blood cells, help maintain healthy bones and other bodily functions, balance body fluids and chemical levels, and retain valuable substances. Graphics demonstrate each of these functions. The narrator reviews the symptoms of kidney failure, and then real patients tell their own experiences of their movement into chronic kidney failure. The program outlines the common causes of chronic kidney failure, including diabetes, glomerulonephritis, hypertension (high blood pressure), polycystic kidney disease, and infections. The remainder of the program outlines each of the treatment options: hemodialysis, peritoneal dialysis, automated peritoneal dialysis (APD), and kidney transplantation. For each type, the program offers live footage of real patients using that treatment, drawings and graphics that demonstrate how the treatment works, and interviews with patients talking about how that treatment affects their lives. The program summarizes the reasons why each treatment option may be appropriate or inappropriate for a specific patient. The program concludes with a list of general guidelines that can help to reduce treatment side effects and with a list of associations to contact for more information.

Bibliography: Multimedia on Polycystic Kidney Disease

The National Library of Medicine is a rich source of information on healthcare-related multimedia productions including slides, computer software, and databases. To access the multimedia database, go to the following Web site: **http://locatorplus.gov/**. Select "Search LOCATORplus." Once in the search area, simply type in polycystic kidney disease (or synonyms). Then, in the option box provided below the search box, select

"Audiovisuals and Computer Files." From there, you can choose to sort results by publication date, author, or relevance. The following multimedia has been indexed on polycystic kidney disease. For more information, follow the hyperlink indicated:

- **Abdominal scanning by ultrasound.** Source: Office of Educational Resources, Univ. of Colo. Medical Ctr.; [made by] University of Colorado Medical Center Television; Year: 1973; Format: Videorecording; [Denver]: The University; [Atlanta: for loan by National Medical Audiovisual Center], 1973

- **Acute renal failure.** Source: University of Michigan, Medical Center, Kidney Foundation, Michigan Dept. of Public Health; produced by University of Michigan, Medical Center, BIomedical Media Production Unit; Year: 1978; Format: Slide; Ann Arbor: The University: [for loan or sale by its Medical Center Media Library], c1978

- **Hand-assisted laparoscopic splenectomy for splenomegaly ; Laparoscopic retroperiton[e]al symphathectomy [i.e. sympathectomy]; Laparoscopic unroofing of symptomatic polycystic kidney disease.** Source: Society American Gastrointestinal Endoscopic; Year: 1999; Format: Videorecording; Woodbury, CT: Distributed by Ciné-Med, [1999]

- **Iatrogenic renal disease.** Source: Benjamin C. Sturgill; Year: 1982; Format: Slide; [New York]: Medcom, c1982

- **Laparoscopic cholecystectomy in a patient with massive polycystic kidneys and polycystic liver disease : a case report.** Source: Steven Wise Unger, Harold M. Unger. A modified laparoscopic cholecystectomy without pneumoperitoneum and with newly d; Year: 1993; Format: Videorecording; [United States]: Society [of] American Gastrointestinal Endoscopic Surgeons, c1993

- **Nutrition and kidney disease.** Source: Emory University School of Medicine; Year: 1973; Format: Videorecording; Atlanta: Georgia Regional Medical Television Network: [for loan or sale by A. W. Calhoun Medical Library, 1973]

- **Polycystic kidney disease and other cystic disorders.** Source: Alexander C. Chester, George E. Schreiner, Harry G. Preuss; Year: 9999; Format: Slide; [New York]: Medcom, c1978-

Vocabulary Builder

Biopsy: The removal and examination, usually microscopic, of tissue from the living body, performed to establish precise diagnosis. [EU]

Cholecystectomy: Surgical removal of the gallbladder. [NIH]

CHAPTER 7. PERIODICALS AND NEWS ON POLYCYSTIC KIDNEY DISEASE

Overview

Keeping up on the news relating to polycystic kidney disease can be challenging. Subscribing to targeted periodicals can be an effective way to stay abreast of recent developments on polycystic kidney disease. Periodicals include newsletters, magazines, and academic journals.

In this chapter, we suggest a number of news sources and present various periodicals that cover polycystic kidney disease beyond and including those which are published by patient associations mentioned earlier. We will first focus on news services, and then on periodicals. News services, press releases, and newsletters generally use more accessible language, so if you do chose to subscribe to one of the more technical periodicals, make sure that it uses language you can easily follow.

News Services & Press Releases

Well before articles show up in newsletters or the popular press, they may appear in the form of a press release or a public relations announcement. One of the simplest ways of tracking press releases on polycystic kidney disease is to search the news wires. News wires are used by professional journalists, and have existed since the invention of the telegraph. Today, there are several major "wires" that are used by companies, universities, and other organizations to announce new medical breakthroughs. In the following sample of sources, we will briefly describe how to access each service. These services only post recent news intended for public viewing.

PR Newswire

Perhaps the broadest of the wires is PR Newswire Association, Inc. To access this archive, simply go to **http://www.prnewswire.com**. Below the search box, select the option "The last 30 days." In the search box, type "polycystic kidney disease" or synonyms. The search results are shown by order of relevance. When reading these press releases, do not forget that the sponsor of the release may be a company or organization that is trying to sell a particular product or therapy. Their views, therefore, may be biased.

Reuters

The Reuters' Medical News database can be very useful in exploring news archives relating to polycystic kidney disease. While some of the listed articles are free to view, others can be purchased for a nominal fee. To access this archive, go to **http://www.reutershealth.com/frame2/arch.html** and search by "polycystic kidney disease" (or synonyms). The following was recently listed in this archive for polycystic kidney disease:

- **Polycystic kidney disease gene product impairs intracellular calcium release**
  Source: Reuters Medical News
  Date: February 19, 2002
  http://www.reuters.gov/archive/2002/02/19/professional/links/20020219scie002.html

- **Gene linked to autosomal recessive polycystic kidney disease**
  Source: Reuters Medical News
  Date: February 05, 2002
  http://www.reuters.gov/archive/2002/02/05/professional/links/20020205scie003.html

- **Mitral valve abnormalities common in patients with polycystic kidney disease**
  Source: Reuters Medical News
  Date: December 28, 2001
  http://www.reuters.gov/archive/2001/12/28/professional/links/20011228epid003.html

- **Defective cilia gene leads to polycystic kidney disease in mouse model**
  Source: Reuters Medical News
  Date: December 12, 2000
  http://www.reuters.gov/archive/2000/12/12/professional/links/20001212scie004.html

- **Concomitant nephrectomy/transplant urged for severe polycystic kidney disease**
  Source: Reuters Medical News
  Date: August 25, 2000
  http://www.reuters.gov/archive/2000/08/25/professional/links/20000825clin001.html

- **Potassium citrate/citric acid ameliorates polycystic kidney disease in rats**
  Source: Reuters Medical News
  Date: July 02, 1998
  http://www.reuters.gov/archive/1998/07/02/professional/links/19980702scie001.html

- **Second Gene For Polycystic Kidney Disease Identified**
  Source: Reuters Medical News
  Date: June 03, 1996
  http://www.reuters.gov/archive/1996/06/03/professional/links/19960603scie002.html

- **Polycystic Kidney Disease Characterized By Apoptosis**
  Source: Reuters Medical News
  Date: July 06, 1995
  http://www.reuters.gov/archive/1995/07/06/professional/links/19950706clin006.html

- **Polycystic Kidney Disease Gene Sequenced**
  Source: Reuters Medical News
  Date: April 03, 1995
  http://www.reuters.gov/archive/1995/04/03/professional/links/19950403clin012.html

The NIH

Within MEDLINEplus, the NIH has made an agreement with the New York Times Syndicate, the AP News Service, and Reuters to deliver news that can be browsed by the public. Search news releases at **http://www.nlm.nih.gov/medlineplus/alphanews_a.html.** MEDLINEplus allows you to browse across an alphabetical index. Or you can search by date at **http://www.nlm.nih.gov/medlineplus/newsbydate.html**. Often, news items are indexed by MEDLINEplus within their search engine.

Business Wire

Business Wire is similar to PR Newswire. To access this archive, simply go to **http://www.businesswire.com**. You can scan the news by industry category or company name.

Internet Wire

Internet Wire is more focused on technology than the other wires. To access this site, go to **http://www.internetwire.com** and use the "Search Archive" option. Type in "polycystic kidney disease" (or synonyms). As this service is oriented to technology, you may wish to search for press releases covering diagnostic procedures or tests that you may have read about.

Search Engines

Free-to-view news can also be found in the news section of your favorite search engines (see the health news page at Yahoo: **http://dir.yahoo.com/Health/News_and_Media/**, or use this Web site's general news search page **http://news.yahoo.com/**. Type in "polycystic kidney disease" (or synonyms). If you know the name of a company that is relevant to polycystic kidney disease, you can go to any stock trading Web site (such as **www.etrade.com**) and search for the company name there. News items across various news sources are reported on indicated hyperlinks.

BBC

Covering news from a more European perspective, the British Broadcasting Corporation (BBC) allows the public free access to their news archive located at **http://www.bbc.co.uk/**. Search by "polycystic kidney disease" (or synonyms).

Newsletter Articles

If you choose not to subscribe to a newsletter, you can nevertheless find references to newsletter articles. We recommend that you use the Combined Health Information Database, while limiting your search criteria to "newsletter articles." Again, you will need to use the "Detailed Search" option. Go to the following hyperlink: **http://chid.nih.gov/detail/detail.html**. Go to the bottom of the search page where "You may refine your search by." Select the dates and language that you prefer. For the format option, select "Newsletter Article."

By making these selections, and typing in "polycystic kidney disease" (or synonyms) into the "For these words:" box, you will only receive results on newsletter articles. You should check back periodically with this database as it is updated every 3 months. The following is a typical result when searching for newsletter articles on polycystic kidney disease:

- **ARPKD: A Quick Review**

  Source: PKD Progress. 16(3): 7. Summer 2001.

  Contact: Available from PKD Foundation. 4901 Main Street, Suite 200, Kansas City, MO 64112-2634. (800) 753-2873. E-mail: pkdcure@pkdcure.org.

  Summary: ARPKD (autosomal recessive polycystic kidney disease) primarily affects, the kidneys (always both) with progressive cysts and the liver with congenital hepatic fibrosis (CHF), which is malformation and progressive scarring of the bile duct system. This brief article reviews ARPKD, its diagnosis and treatment. The author notes that because of continually improved mechanical ventilation, neonate support, control of systemic and portal hypertension, management of ESRD, and transplantation, the ARPKD population is living longer into adulthood. Unfortunately, 30 to 50 percent of infants with ARPKD die at birthor shortly thereafter, usually as a result of underdeveloped lungs and pulmonary complications. Almost everyone with ARPKD is diagnosed during infancy or childhood; however, the first signs of the disease vary greatly. Approximately 30 percent of the infants experience failure-to-thrive, although the exact cause is unknown. Hypertension (high blood pressure) is thought to be a factor in progression of renal deterioration, and without aggressive treatment, severe hypertension can be life threatening. The same inherited defect that affects the kidneys occurs in the liver, but the two organs react differently with great variability of onset and severity of clinical symptoms. Even for symptomatic individuals, synthetic liver function generally is preserved, as it usually continues to excrete, produce, and regulate hormones and chemicals normally.

- **Anemia-Related Fatigue: Feeling Tired Isn't Always Normal**

  Source: PKR Progress. 15(3): 10. Fall-Winter 2000.

Contact: PKD Foundation. 4901 Main Street, Suite 200, Kansas City, MO 64112-2634. (800) 753-2873. E-mail: pkdcure@pkdcure.org.

Summary: This article from a newsletter for patients with polycystic kidney disease (PKD) explores the problem of anemia related fatigue in patients with kidney diseases. The author notes that since basic treatments are available for PKD, health care providers and researchers are now turning their attention to quality of life medical issues such as anemia. Anemia develops in virtually all patients with renal failure during the course of their disease. Health care providers now know that by intervening earlier in the disease process (in patients with chronic kidney disease who are not yet on dialysis), patients can realize a number of benefits and enhance their overall well being. The kidneys produce about 90 percent of the body's supply of the hormone erythropoietin (EPO); EPO is a major catalyst in the production of red blood cells in the bone marrow, so a reduction in EPO due to kidney disease usually results in fewer red blood cells and insufficient oxygen reaching the body tissues. The author explains the two primary diagnostic tests used to check for anemia, hematocrit (HCT) and hemoglobin. Anemia related fatigue is often described as a total lack of energy or debilitating exhaustion that can last days, weeks, or months. Fatigue can also have mental and emotional effects. The author cautions that because of its gradual onset and insidious nature, fatigue is often overlooked, underrecognized, and undertreated. Readers are encouraged to work with their physicians to address any problems or symptoms of fatigue.

- **Genes Behaving Badly**

Source: PKR Progress. 13(2): 4-5, 17. Spring 1998.

Contact: Available from Polycystic Kidney Research Foundation. 4901 Main Street, Suite 200, Kansas City, MO 64112-2634. (800) 753-2873 or (816) 931-2600. Fax (816) 931-8655.

Summary: One of the striking features of polycystic kidney disease (PKD) is the variability with which it affects people. Some individuals develop a modest number of cysts throughout their lifetime and do not even know they are affected by the disorder. Others develop a massive amount of cysts on their kidneys and reach renal failure at a young age. This article summarizes recent data from studies that are attempting to identify the factors and determine the processes that account for these differences. The author discusses three areas of study: interfamilial variability, intrafamilial variability, and intraindividual variability. The author describes how differences in the type of PKD or the influence of genetic modifiers may explain different disease presentations in different families; however, these differences do not cover variability between individuals. Careful analysis of early cystic kidneys reveals that only a small subset of tubules develop cysts. Researchers are trying to determine how the cells that go on to become cysts differ from those that do not. The author describes the focal nature of renal cyst formation and the molecular basis of focal cyst formation. A sidebar urges readers who are interested in participating in research studies to contact the study coordinator (telephone number provided). 2 figures.

Academic Periodicals covering Polycystic Kidney Disease

Academic periodicals can be a highly technical yet valuable source of information on polycystic kidney disease. We have compiled the following list of periodicals known to publish articles relating to polycystic kidney disease and which are currently indexed within the National Library of Medicine's PubMed database (follow hyperlinks to view more information, summaries, etc., for each). In addition to these sources, to keep current on articles written on polycystic kidney disease published by any of the periodicals listed below, you can simply follow the hyperlink indicated or go to the following Web site: **www.ncbi.nlm.nih.gov/pubmed**. Type the periodical's name into the search box to find the latest studies published.

If you want complete details about the historical contents of a periodical, you can also visit **http://www.ncbi.nlm.nih.gov/entrez/jrbrowser.cgi**. Here, type in the name of the journal or its abbreviation, and you will receive an index of published articles. At **http://locatorplus.gov/** you can retrieve more indexing information on medical periodicals (e.g. the name of the publisher). Select the button "Search LOCATORplus." Then type in the name of the journal and select the advanced search option "Journal Title Search." The following is a sample of periodicals which publish articles on polycystic kidney disease:

- **American Journal of Kidney Diseases : the Official Journal of the National Kidney Foundation. (Am J Kidney Dis)**
  http://www.ncbi.nlm.nih.gov/entrez/jrbrowser.cgi?field=0&regexp=American+Journal+of+Kidney+Diseases+:+the+Official+Journal+of+the+National+Kidney+Foundation&dispmax=20&dispstart=0

- **Kidney International. (Kidney Int)**
  http://www.ncbi.nlm.nih.gov/entrez/jrbrowser.cgi?field=0&regexp=Ki
  dney+International&dispmax=20&dispstart=0

- **Nephrology, Dialysis, Transplantation : Official Publication of the European Dialysis and Transplant Association - European Renal Association. (Nephrol Dial Transplant)**
  http://www.ncbi.nlm.nih.gov/entrez/jrbrowser.cgi?field=0&regexp=Ne
  phrology,+Dialysis,+Transplantation+:+Official+Publication+of+the+Eur
  opean+Dialysis+and+Transplant+Association+-
  +European+Renal+Association&dispmax=20&dispstart=0

Vocabulary Builder

Anemia: A reduction in the number of circulating erythrocytes or in the quantity of hemoglobin. [NIH]

Hematocrit: Measurement of the volume of packed red cells in a blood specimen by centrifugation. The procedure is performed using a tube with graduated markings or with automated blood cell counters. It is used as an indicator of erythrocyte status in disease. For example, anemia shows a low hematocrit, polycythemia, high values. [NIH]

Ventilation: 1. in respiratory physiology, the process of exchange of air between the lungs and the ambient air. Pulmonary ventilation (usually measured in litres per minute) refers to the total exchange, whereas alveolar ventilation refers to the effective ventilation of the alveoli, in which gas exchange with the blood takes place. 2. in psychiatry, verbalization of one's emotional problems. [EU]

CHAPTER 8. PHYSICIAN GUIDELINES AND DATABASES

Overview

Doctors and medical researchers rely on a number of information sources to help patients with their conditions. Many will subscribe to journals or newsletters published by their professional associations or refer to specialized textbooks or clinical guides published for the medical profession. In this chapter, we focus on databases and Internet-based guidelines created or written for this professional audience.

NIH Guidelines

For the more common diseases, The National Institutes of Health publish guidelines that are frequently consulted by physicians. Publications are typically written by one or more of the various NIH Institutes. For physician guidelines, commonly referred to as "clinical" or "professional" guidelines, you can visit the following Institutes:

- Office of the Director (OD); guidelines consolidated across agencies available at **http://www.nih.gov/health/consumer/conkey.htm**

- National Institute of General Medical Sciences (NIGMS); fact sheets available at **http://www.nigms.nih.gov/news/facts/**

- National Library of Medicine (NLM); extensive encyclopedia (A.D.A.M., Inc.) with guidelines:
  http://www.nlm.nih.gov/medlineplus/healthtopics.html

- National Institute of Diabetes and Digestive and Kidney Diseases (NIDDK); guidelines available at
  http://www.niddk.nih.gov/health/health.htm

NIH Databases

In addition to the various Institutes of Health that publish professional guidelines, the NIH has designed a number of databases for professionals.[25] Physician-oriented resources provide a wide variety of information related to the biomedical and health sciences, both past and present. The format of these resources varies. Searchable databases, bibliographic citations, full text articles (when available), archival collections, and images are all available. The following are referenced by the National Library of Medicine:[26]

- **Bioethics:** Access to published literature on the ethical, legal and public policy issues surrounding healthcare and biomedical research. This information is provided in conjunction with the Kennedy Institute of Ethics located at Georgetown University, Washington, D.C.: **http://www.nlm.nih.gov/databases/databases_bioethics.html**

- **HIV/AIDS Resources:** Describes various links and databases dedicated to HIV/AIDS research: **http://www.nlm.nih.gov/pubs/factsheets/aidsinfs.html**

- **NLM Online Exhibitions:** Describes "Exhibitions in the History of Medicine": **http://www.nlm.nih.gov/exhibition/exhibition.html**. Additional resources for historical scholarship in medicine: **http://www.nlm.nih.gov/hmd/hmd.html**

- **Biotechnology Information:** Access to public databases. The National Center for Biotechnology Information conducts research in computational biology, develops software tools for analyzing genome data, and disseminates biomedical information for the better understanding of molecular processes affecting human health and disease: **http://www.ncbi.nlm.nih.gov/**

- **Population Information:** The National Library of Medicine provides access to worldwide coverage of population, family planning, and related health issues, including family planning technology and programs, fertility, and population law and policy: **http://www.nlm.nih.gov/databases/databases_population.html**

- **Cancer Information:** Access to caner-oriented databases: **http://www.nlm.nih.gov/databases/databases_cancer.html**

---

[25] Remember, for the general public, the National Library of Medicine recommends the databases referenced in MEDLINE*plus* (**http://medlineplus.gov/** or **http://www.nlm.nih.gov/medlineplus/databases.html**).
[26] See **http://www.nlm.nih.gov/databases/databases.html**.

- **Profiles in Science:** Offering the archival collections of prominent twentieth-century biomedical scientists to the public through modern digital technology: **http://www.profiles.nlm.nih.gov/**

- **Chemical Information:** Provides links to various chemical databases and references: **http://sis.nlm.nih.gov/Chem/ChemMain.html**

- **Clinical Alerts:** Reports the release of findings from the NIH-funded clinical trials where such release could significantly affect morbidity and mortality: **http://www.nlm.nih.gov/databases/alerts/clinical_alerts.html**

- **Space Life Sciences:** Provides links and information to space-based research (including NASA):
  http://www.nlm.nih.gov/databases/databases_space.html

- **MEDLINE:** Bibliographic database covering the fields of medicine, nursing, dentistry, veterinary medicine, the healthcare system, and the pre-clinical sciences:
  http://www.nlm.nih.gov/databases/databases_medline.html

- **Toxicology and Environmental Health Information (TOXNET):** Databases covering toxicology and environmental health:
  http://sis.nlm.nih.gov/Tox/ToxMain.html

- **Visible Human Interface:** Anatomically detailed, three-dimensional representations of normal male and female human bodies:
  http://www.nlm.nih.gov/research/visible/visible_human.html

While all of the above references may be of interest to physicians who study and treat polycystic kidney disease, the following are particularly noteworthy.

The Combined Health Information Database

A comprehensive source of information on clinical guidelines written for professionals is the Combined Health Information Database. You will need to limit your search to "Brochure/Pamphlet," "Fact Sheet," or "Information Package" and polycystic kidney disease using the "Detailed Search" option. Go to the following hyperlink: **http://chid.nih.gov/detail/detail.html**. To find associations, use the drop boxes at the bottom of the search page where "You may refine your search by." For the publication date, select "All Years," select your preferred language, and the format option "Fact Sheet." By making these selections and typing "polycystic kidney disease" (or synonyms) into the "For these words:" box above, you will only receive results on fact sheets dealing with polycystic kidney disease. The following is a sample result:

- **Facts About Kidney Diseases and Their Treatment**

  Source: Rockville, MD: American Kidney Fund. 1999. 13 p.

  Contact: Available from American Kidney Fund. 6110 Executive Boulevard, Suite 1010, Rockville, MD 20852. (800) 638-8299 or (301) 881-3052. Fax (301) 881-0898. E-mail: helpline@akfinc.org. Website: www.akfinc.org. Price: $0.30 plus shipping and handling.

  Summary: This brochure from the American Kidney Fund (AKF) informs the public about the signs, symptoms, and methods of treatment for various kidney diseases. The brochure begins by reviewing the anatomy and physiology of the kidneys, whose primary job is to remove waste from the blood and eliminate it in the urine. The kidneys also keep the right amount of fluid in the body by making more urine when there is too much fluid. Kidney disease is actually a catch all term that includes diseases ranging from urinary tract infections, to kidney stones, to more serious disorders such as polycystic kidney disease and glomerulonephritis. Many kidney diseases can be effectively treated if diagnosed in the early stages. The brochure stresses that high blood pressure (hypertension) can cause kidney disease and must be monitored and treated. The brochure reviews the more common diseases of the kidneys, including kidney stones, pyelonephritis (inflammation of kidney tissue due to infection), nephrosis (a condition in which the kidneys remove too much protein from the blood), glomerulonephritis (inflammation of the thin walled capillaries where filtration takes place), polycystic kidney disease, and end stage renal disease (ESRD). The brochure details the treatments available for ESRD, including hemodialysis, peritoneal dialysis, and transplantation. The brochure concludes with a summary of facts to remember about kidney diseases, reiterating the importance of controlling high blood pressure. The back cover of the brochure briefly notes the goals and activities of the American Kidney Fund. 4 figures.

- **Your Kidneys: Master Chemists of the Body**

  Source: New York, NY: National Kidney Foundation. 1996. 14 p.

  Contact: National Kidney Foundation. 30 East 33rd Street, New York, NY 10016. (800) 622-9010. Website: www.kidney.org. Price: Single copy free; bulk copies available.

  Summary: The schematic drawings of the urinary system in this booklet describe the location of the kidneys in the body and the kidney filtering system. Types and causes of kidney disease are also discussed including diabetes, high blood pressure, glomerulonephritis, polycystic kidney disease, kidney stones, urinary tract infections, and congenital diseases. The warning signs of kidney disease and the treatments available for advanced kidney failure are considered briefly.

The NLM Gateway[27]

The NLM (National Library of Medicine) Gateway is a Web-based system that lets users search simultaneously in multiple retrieval systems at the U.S. National Library of Medicine (NLM). It allows users of NLM services to initiate searches from one Web interface, providing "one-stop searching" for many of NLM's information resources or databases.[28] One target audience for the Gateway is the Internet user who is new to NLM's online resources and does not know what information is available or how best to search for it. This audience may include physicians and other healthcare providers, researchers, librarians, students, and, increasingly, patients, their families, and the public.[29] To use the NLM Gateway, simply go to the search site at **http://gateway.nlm.nih.gov/gw/Cmd**. Type "polycystic kidney disease" (or synonyms) into the search box and click "Search." The results will be presented in a tabular form, indicating the number of references in each database category.

---

[27] Adapted from NLM: **http://gateway.nlm.nih.gov/gw/Cmd?Overview.x**.

[28] The NLM Gateway is currently being developed by the Lister Hill National Center for Biomedical Communications (LHNCBC) at the National Library of Medicine (NLM) of the National Institutes of Health (NIH).

[29] Other users may find the Gateway useful for an overall search of NLM's information resources. Some searchers may locate what they need immediately, while others will utilize the Gateway as an adjunct tool to other NLM search services such as PubMed® and MEDLINEplus®. The Gateway connects users with multiple NLM retrieval systems while also providing a search interface for its own collections. These collections include various types of information that do not logically belong in PubMed, LOCATORplus, or other established NLM retrieval systems (e.g., meeting announcements and pre-1966 journal citations). The Gateway will provide access to the information found in an increasing number of NLM retrieval systems in several phases.

Results Summary

Category	Items Found
Journal Articles	3667
Books / Periodicals / Audio Visual	See Details
Consumer Health	18
Meeting Abstracts	0
Other Collections	0
Total	3685

HSTAT[30]

HSTAT is a free, Web-based resource that provides access to full-text documents used in healthcare decision-making.[31] HSTAT's audience includes healthcare providers, health service researchers, policy makers, insurance companies, consumers, and the information professionals who serve these groups. HSTAT provides access to a wide variety of publications, including clinical practice guidelines, quick-reference guides for clinicians, consumer health brochures, evidence reports and technology assessments from the Agency for Healthcare Research and Quality (AHRQ), as well as AHRQ's Put Prevention Into Practice.[32] Simply search by "polycystic kidney disease" (or synonyms) at the following Web site: **http://text.nlm.nih.gov**.

Coffee Break: Tutorials for Biologists[33]

Some patients may wish to have access to a general healthcare site that takes a scientific view of the news and covers recent breakthroughs in biology that may one day assist physicians in developing treatments. To this end, we

[30] Adapted from HSTAT: **http://www.nlm.nih.gov/pubs/factsheets/hstat.html**

[31] The HSTAT URL is **http://hstat.nlm.nih.gov/**.

[32] Other important documents in HSTAT include: the National Institutes of Health (NIH) Consensus Conference Reports and Technology Assessment Reports; the HIV/AIDS Treatment Information Service (ATIS) resource documents; the Substance Abuse and Mental Health Services Administration's Center for Substance Abuse Treatment (SAMHSA/CSAT) Treatment Improvement Protocols (TIP) and Center for Substance Abuse Prevention (SAMHSA/CSAP) Prevention Enhancement Protocols System (PEPS); the Public Health Service (PHS) Preventive Services Task Force's *Guide to Clinical Preventive Services*; the independent, nonfederal Task Force on Community Services *Guide to Community Preventive Services*; and the Health Technology Advisory Committee (HTAC) of the Minnesota Health Care Commission (MHCC) health technology evaluations.

[33] Adapted from **http://www.ncbi.nlm.nih.gov/Coffeebreak/Archive/FAQ.html**

recommend "Coffee Break," a collection of short reports on recent biological discoveries. Each report incorporates interactive tutorials that demonstrate how bioinformatics tools are used as a part of the research process. Currently, all Coffee Breaks are written by NCBI staff.[34] Each report is about 400 words and is usually based on a discovery reported in one or more articles from recently published, peer-reviewed literature.[35] This site has new articles every few weeks, so it can be considered an online magazine of sorts, and intended for general background information. You can access the Coffee Break Web site at **http://www.ncbi.nlm.nih.gov/Coffeebreak/**.

Other Commercial Databases

In addition to resources maintained by official agencies, other databases exist that are commercial ventures addressing medical professionals. Here are a few examples that may interest you:

- **CliniWeb International:** Index and table of contents to selected clinical information on the Internet; see **http://www.ohsu.edu/cliniweb/**.

- **Image Engine:** Multimedia electronic medical record system that integrates a wide range of digitized clinical images with textual data stored in the University of Pittsburgh Medical Center's MARS electronic medical record system; see the following Web site: **http://www.cml.upmc.edu/cml/imageengine/imageEngine.html**.

- **Medical World Search:** Searches full text from thousands of selected medical sites on the Internet; see **http://www.mwsearch.com/**.

- **MedWeaver:** Prototype system that allows users to search differential diagnoses for any list of signs and symptoms, to search medical literature, and to explore relevant Web sites; see **http://www.med.virginia.edu/~wmd4n/medweaver.html**.

- **Metaphrase:** Middleware component intended for use by both caregivers and medical records personnel. It converts the informal language generally used by caregivers into terms from formal, controlled vocabularies; see **http://www.lexical.com/Metaphrase.html**.

---

[34] The figure that accompanies each article is frequently supplied by an expert external to NCBI, in which case the source of the figure is cited. The result is an interactive tutorial that tells a biological story.

[35] After a brief introduction that sets the work described into a broader context, the report focuses on how a molecular understanding can provide explanations of observed biology and lead to therapies for diseases. Each vignette is accompanied by a figure and hypertext links that lead to a series of pages that interactively show how NCBI tools and resources are used in the research process.

The Genome Project and Polycystic Kidney Disease

With all the discussion in the press about the Human Genome Project, it is only natural that physicians, researchers, and patients want to know about how human genes relate to polycystic kidney disease. In the following section, we will discuss databases and references used by physicians and scientists who work in this area.

Online Mendelian Inheritance in Man (OMIM)

The Online Mendelian Inheritance in Man (OMIM) database is a catalog of human genes and genetic disorders authored and edited by Dr. Victor A. McKusick and his colleagues at Johns Hopkins and elsewhere. OMIM was developed for the World Wide Web by the National Center for Biotechnology Information (NCBI).[36] The database contains textual information, pictures, and reference information. It also contains copious links to NCBI's Entrez database of MEDLINE articles and sequence information.

Go to **http://www.ncbi.nlm.nih.gov/Omim/searchomim.html** to search the database. Type "polycystic kidney disease" (or synonyms) in the search box, and click "Submit Search." If too many results appear, you can narrow the search by adding the word "clinical." Each report will have additional links to related research and databases. By following these links, especially the link titled "Database Links," you will be exposed to numerous specialized databases that are largely used by the scientific community. These databases are overly technical and seldom used by the general public, but offer an abundance of information. The following is an example of the results you can obtain from the OMIM for polycystic kidney disease:

- **Polycystic Kidney Disease 1**
  Web site: http://www.ncbi.nlm.nih.gov/htbin-
  post/Omim/dispmim?601313

- **Polycystic Kidney Disease 2**
  Web site: http://www.ncbi.nlm.nih.gov/htbin-
  post/Omim/dispmim?173910

---

[36] Adapted from **http://www.ncbi.nlm.nih.gov/**. Established in 1988 as a national resource for molecular biology information, NCBI creates public databases, conducts research in computational biology, develops software tools for analyzing genome data, and disseminates biomedical information--all for the better understanding of molecular processes affecting human health and disease.

- **Polycystic Kidney Disease 2-like 1**
  Web site: http://www.ncbi.nlm.nih.gov/htbin-post/Omim/dispmim?604532

- **Polycystic Kidney Disease 2-like 2**
  Web site: http://www.ncbi.nlm.nih.gov/htbin-post/Omim/dispmim?604669

- **Polycystic Kidney Disease 3, Autosomal Dominant**
  Web site: http://www.ncbi.nlm.nih.gov/htbin-post/Omim/dispmim?600666

- **Polycystic Kidney Disease and Sea Urchin Rej Homolog-like**
  Web site: http://www.ncbi.nlm.nih.gov/htbin-post/Omim/dispmim?604670

- **Polycystic Kidney Disease, Autosomal Recessive**
  Web site: http://www.ncbi.nlm.nih.gov/htbin-post/Omim/dispmim?263200

- **Polycystic Kidney Disease, Autosomal Recessive**
  Web site: http://www.ncbi.nlm.nih.gov/htbin-post/Omim/dispmim?600595

- **Polycystic Kidney Disease, Infantile Severe, with Tuberous Sclerosis**
  Web site: http://www.ncbi.nlm.nih.gov/htbin-post/Omim/dispmim?600273

- **Polycystic Kidney Disease, Potter Type I, with Microbrachycephaly, Hypertelorism, and Brachymelia**
  Web site: http://www.ncbi.nlm.nih.gov/htbin-post/Omim/dispmim?263210

Genes and Disease (NCBI - Map)

The Genes and Disease database is produced by the National Center for Biotechnology Information of the National Library of Medicine at the National Institutes of Health. Go to **http://www.ncbi.nlm.nih.gov/disease/**, and browse the system pages to have a full view of important conditions linked to human genes. Since this site is regularly updated, you may wish to re-visit it from time to time. The following systems and associated disorders are addressed:

- **Immune System:** Fights invaders.
  Examples: Asthma, autoimmune polyglandular syndrome, Crohn's disease, DiGeorge syndrome, familial Mediterranean fever,

immunodeficiency with Hyper-IgM, severe combined immunodeficiency.
Web site: **http://www.ncbi.nlm.nih.gov/disease/Immune.html**

- **Muscle and Bone:** Movement and growth.
  Examples: Duchenne muscular dystrophy, Ellis-van Creveld syndrome,
  Marfan syndrome, myotonic dystrophy, spinal muscular atrophy.
  Web site: **http://www.ncbi.nlm.nih.gov/disease/Muscle.html**

- **Signals:** Cellular messages.
  Examples: Ataxia telangiectasia, Baldness, Cockayne syndrome,
  Glaucoma, SRY: sex determination, Tuberous sclerosis, Waardenburg
  syndrome, Werner syndrome.
  Web site: **http://www.ncbi.nlm.nih.gov/disease/Signals.html**

- **Transporters:** Pumps and channels.
  Examples: Cystic Fibrosis, deafness, diastrophic dysplasia, Hemophilia
  A, long-QT syndrome, Menkes syndrome, Pendred syndrome, polycystic
  kidney disease, sickle cell anemia, Wilson's disease, Zellweger syndrome.
  Web site: **http://www.ncbi.nlm.nih.gov/disease/Transporters.html**

Entrez

Entrez is a search and retrieval system that integrates several linked
databases at the National Center for Biotechnology Information (NCBI).
These databases include nucleotide sequences, protein sequences,
macromolecular structures, whole genomes, and MEDLINE through
PubMed. Entrez provides access to the following databases:

- **PubMed:** Biomedical literature (PubMed),
  Web site: **http://www.ncbi.nlm.nih.gov/entrez/query.fcgi?db=PubMed**

- **Nucleotide Sequence Database (Genbank):**
  Web site:
  http://www.ncbi.nlm.nih.gov/entrez/query.fcgi?db=Nucleotide

- **Protein Sequence Database:**
  Web site: **http://www.ncbi.nlm.nih.gov/entrez/query.fcgi?db=Protein**

- **Structure:** Three-dimensional macromolecular structures,
  Web site: **http://www.ncbi.nlm.nih.gov/entrez/query.fcgi?db=Structure**

- **Genome:** Complete genome assemblies,
  Web site: **http://www.ncbi.nlm.nih.gov/entrez/query.fcgi?db=Genome**

- **PopSet:** Population study data sets,
  Web site: **http://www.ncbi.nlm.nih.gov/entrez/query.fcgi?db=Popset**

- **OMIM:** Online Mendelian Inheritance in Man,
  Web site: **http://www.ncbi.nlm.nih.gov/entrez/query.fcgi?db=OMIM**

- **Taxonomy:** Organisms in GenBank,
  Web site:
  http://www.ncbi.nlm.nih.gov/entrez/query.fcgi?db=Taxonomy

- **Books:** Online books,
  Web site: **http://www.ncbi.nlm.nih.gov/entrez/query.fcgi?db=books**

- **ProbeSet:** Gene Expression Omnibus (GEO),
  Web site: **http://www.ncbi.nlm.nih.gov/entrez/query.fcgi?db=geo**

- **3D Domains:** Domains from Entrez Structure,
  Web site: **http://www.ncbi.nlm.nih.gov/entrez/query.fcgi?db=geo**

- **NCBI's Protein Sequence Information Survey Results:**
  Web site: **http://www.ncbi.nlm.nih.gov/About/proteinsurvey/**

To access the Entrez system at the National Center for Biotechnology Information, go to **http://www.ncbi.nlm.nih.gov/entrez/**, and then select the database that you would like to search. The databases available are listed in the drop box next to "Search." In the box next to "for," enter "polycystic kidney disease" (or synonyms) and click "Go."

Jablonski's Multiple Congenital Anomaly/Mental Retardation (MCA/MR) Syndromes Database[37]

This online resource can be quite useful. It has been developed to facilitate the identification and differentiation of syndromic entities. Special attention is given to the type of information that is usually limited or completely omitted in existing reference sources due to space limitations of the printed form.

At **http://www.nlm.nih.gov/mesh/jablonski/syndrome_toc/toc_a.html** you can also search across syndromes using an alphabetical index. You can also search at **http://www.nlm.nih.gov/mesh/jablonski/syndrome_db.html**.

---

[37] Adapted from the National Library of Medicine:
http://www.nlm.nih.gov/mesh/jablonski/about_syndrome.html.

The Genome Database[38]

Established at Johns Hopkins University in Baltimore, Maryland in 1990, the Genome Database (GDB) is the official central repository for genomic mapping data resulting from the Human Genome Initiative. In the spring of 1999, the Bioinformatics Supercomputing Centre (BiSC) at the Hospital for Sick Children in Toronto, Ontario assumed the management of GDB. The Human Genome Initiative is a worldwide research effort focusing on structural analysis of human DNA to determine the location and sequence of the estimated 100,000 human genes. In support of this project, GDB stores and curates data generated by researchers worldwide who are engaged in the mapping effort of the Human Genome Project (HGP). GDB's mission is to provide scientists with an encyclopedia of the human genome which is continually revised and updated to reflect the current state of scientific knowledge. Although GDB has historically focused on gene mapping, its focus will broaden as the Genome Project moves from mapping to sequence, and finally, to functional analysis.

To access the GDB, simply go to the following hyperlink: **http://www.gdb.org/**. Search "All Biological Data" by "Keyword." Type "polycystic kidney disease" (or synonyms) into the search box, and review the results. If more than one word is used in the search box, then separate each one with the word "and" or "or" (using "or" might be useful when using synonyms). This database is extremely technical as it was created for specialists. The articles are the results which are the most accessible to non-professionals and often listed under the heading "Citations." The contact names are also accessible to non-professionals.

Specialized References

The following books are specialized references written for professionals interested in polycystic kidney disease (sorted alphabetically by title, hyperlinks provide rankings, information, and reviews at Amazon.com):

- **Adult and Pediatric Urology (3-Volume Set) (Includes a Card to Return to Receive the Free CD-ROM)** by Jay Y. Gillenwater, M.D. (Editor), et al; Hardcover - 2828 pages, 4th edition (January 15, 2002), Lippincott, Williams & Wilkins Publishers; ISBN: 0781732204; **http://www.amazon.com/exec/obidos/ASIN/0781732204/icongroupinterna**

---

[38] Adapted from the Genome Database: **http://gdbwww.gdb.org/gdb/aboutGDB.html#mission**.

- **Campbell's Urology (4-Volume Set)** by Meredith F. Campbell (Editor), et al; Hardcover, 8th edition (May 15, 2002), W B Saunders Co; ISBN: 0721690580;
http://www.amazon.com/exec/obidos/ASIN/0721690580/icongroupinterna

- **Clinical Manual of Urology** by Philip M. Hanno, M.D. (Editor), et al; Paperback - 924 pages, 3rd edition (May 2, 2001), McGraw-Hill Professional Publishing; ISBN: 0071362010;
http://www.amazon.com/exec/obidos/ASIN/0071362010/icongroupinterna

- **Comprehensive Urology** by George Weiss O'Reilly; Hardcover - 724 pages, 1st edition (January 15, 2001), Elsevier Science, Health Science Division; ISBN: 0723429499;
http://www.amazon.com/exec/obidos/ASIN/0723429499/icongroupinterna

- **Manual of Urology: Diagnosis & Therapy** by Mike B. Siroky (Editor), et al; Spiral-bound - 362 pages, 2nd spiral edition (October 15, 1999), Lippincott, Williams & Wilkins Publishers; ISBN: 078171785X;
http://www.amazon.com/exec/obidos/ASIN/078171785X/icongroupinterna

- **The Scientific Basis of Urology** by A.R. Mundy (Editor), et al; 531 pages - 1st edition (March 15, 1999), Isis Medical Media; ISBN: 1899066217;
http://www.amazon.com/exec/obidos/ASIN/1899066217/icongroupinterna

- **Smith's General Urology** by Emil A. Tanagho (Editor), et al; Paperback - 888 pages, 15th edition (January 21, 2000), McGraw-Hill Professional Publishing; ISBN: 0838586074;
http://www.amazon.com/exec/obidos/ASIN/0838586074/icongroupinterna

- **Urology (House Officer Series)** by Michael T. MacFarlane, M.D.; Paperback - 3rd edition (January 2001), Lippincott, Williams & Wilkins Publishers; ISBN: 0781731461;
http://www.amazon.com/exec/obidos/ASIN/0781731461/icongroupinterna

- **Urology for Primary Care Physicians** by Unyime O. Nseyo (Editor), et al; Hardcover - 399 pages, 1st edition (July 15, 1999), W B Saunders Co; ISBN: 0721671489;
http://www.amazon.com/exec/obidos/ASIN/0721671489/icongroupinterna

Vocabulary Builder

Hypertelorism: Abnormal increase in the interorbital distance due to overdevelopment of the lesser wings of the sphenoid. [NIH]

Inflammation: A pathological process characterized by injury or destruction of tissues caused by a variety of cytologic and chemical reactions. It is usually manifested by typical signs of pain, heat, redness, swelling, and loss of function. [NIH]

Nephrosis: Descriptive histopathologic term for renal disease without an inflammatory component. [NIH]

Pyelonephritis: Inflammation of the kidney and its pelvis, beginning in the interstitium and rapidly extending to involve the tubules, glomeruli, and blood vessels; due to bacterial infection. [EU]

CHAPTER 9. DISSERTATIONS ON POLYCYSTIC KIDNEY DISEASE

Overview

University researchers are active in studying almost all known diseases. The result of research is often published in the form of Doctoral or Master's dissertations. You should understand, therefore, that applied diagnostic procedures and/or therapies can take many years to develop after the thesis that proposed the new technique or approach was written.

In this chapter, we will give you a bibliography on recent dissertations relating to polycystic kidney disease. You can read about these in more detail using the Internet or your local medical library. We will also provide you with information on how to use the Internet to stay current on dissertations.

Dissertations on Polycystic Kidney Disease

ProQuest Digital Dissertations is the largest archive of academic dissertations available. From this archive, we have compiled the following list covering dissertations devoted to polycystic kidney disease. You will see that the information provided includes the dissertation's title, its author, and the author's institution. To read more about the following, simply use the Internet address indicated. The following covers recent dissertations dealing with polycystic kidney disease:

- **Dietary Fat Level and Source Alter Renal Disease Progression in Animal Models of Polycystic Kidney Disease** by Lu, Jing; Phd from Texas Woman's University, 2000, 105 pages
http://wwwlib.umi.com/dissertations/fullcit/9976863

- **Effects of a Creatine/glutamine Dietary Supplement and Moderate Aerobic Exercise on Kidney Disease Progression in a Male Animal Model of Polycystic Kidney Disease** by Cribbs, Ciaran; Ms from Texas Woman's University, 2000, 102 pages
http://wwwlib.umi.com/dissertations/fullcit/1402182

- **Egf and C-myc in Cpk-induced Murine Autosomal Recessive Polycystic Kidney Disease** by Ricker, Justin Lynn; Phd from University of Kansas, 2000, 192 pages
http://wwwlib.umi.com/dissertations/fullcit/9988930

Keeping Current

As previously mentioned, an effective way to stay current on dissertations dedicated to polycystic kidney disease is to use the database called *ProQuest Digital Dissertations* via the Internet, located at the following Web address: **http://wwwlib.umi.com/dissertations.** The site allows you to freely access the last two years of citations and abstracts. Ask your medical librarian if the library has full and unlimited access to this database. From the library, you should be able to do more complete searches than with the limited 2-year access available to the general public.

Vocabulary Builder

Aerobic: 1. having molecular oxygen present. 2. growing, living, or occurring in the presence of molecular oxygen. 3. requiring oxygen for respiration. [EU]

Creatine: An amino acid that occurs in vertebrate tissues and in urine. In muscle tissue, creatine generally occurs as phosphocreatine. Creatine is excreted as creatinine in the urine. [NIH]

Glutamine: A non-essential amino acid present abundantly throught the body and is involved in many metabolic processes. It is synthesized from glutamic acid and ammonia. It is the principal carrier of nitrogen in the body and is an important energy source for many cells. [NIH]

PART III. APPENDICES

ABOUT PART III

Part III is a collection of appendices on general medical topics which may be of interest to patients with polycystic kidney disease and related conditions.

APPENDIX A. RESEARCHING YOUR MEDICATIONS

Overview

There are a number of sources available on new or existing medications which could be prescribed to patients with polycystic kidney disease. While a number of hard copy or CD-Rom resources are available to patients and physicians for research purposes, a more flexible method is to use Internet-based databases. In this chapter, we will begin with a general overview of medications. We will then proceed to outline official recommendations on how you should view your medications. You may also want to research medications that you are currently taking for other conditions as they may interact with medications for polycystic kidney disease. Research can give you information on the side effects, interactions, and limitations of prescription drugs used in the treatment of polycystic kidney disease. Broadly speaking, there are two sources of information on approved medications: public sources and private sources. We will emphasize free-to-use public sources.

Your Medications: The Basics[39]

The Agency for Health Care Research and Quality has published extremely useful guidelines on how you can best participate in the medication aspects of polycystic kidney disease. Taking medicines is not always as simple as swallowing a pill. It can involve many steps and decisions each day. The AHCRQ recommends that patients with polycystic kidney disease take part in treatment decisions. Do not be afraid to ask questions and talk about your concerns. By taking a moment to ask questions early, you may avoid problems later. Here are some points to cover each time a new medicine is prescribed:

- Ask about all parts of your treatment, including diet changes, exercise, and medicines.

- Ask about the risks and benefits of each medicine or other treatment you might receive.

- Ask how often you or your doctor will check for side effects from a given medication.

Do not hesitate to ask what is important to you about your medicines. You may want a medicine with the fewest side effects, or the fewest doses to take each day. You may care most about cost, or how the medicine might affect how you live or work. Or, you may want the medicine your doctor believes will work the best. Telling your doctor will help him or her select the best treatment for you.

Do not be afraid to "bother" your doctor with your concerns and questions about medications for polycystic kidney disease. You can also talk to a nurse or a pharmacist. They can help you better understand your treatment plan. Feel free to bring a friend or family member with you when you visit your doctor. Talking over your options with someone you trust can help you make better choices, especially if you are not feeling well. Specifically, ask your doctor the following:

- The name of the medicine and what it is supposed to do.

- How and when to take the medicine, how much to take, and for how long.

- What food, drinks, other medicines, or activities you should avoid while taking the medicine.

- What side effects the medicine may have, and what to do if they occur.

---

[39] This section is adapted from AHCRQ: **http://www.ahcpr.gov/consumer/ncpiebro.htm**.

- If you can get a refill, and how often.

- About any terms or directions you do not understand.

- What to do if you miss a dose.

- If there is written information you can take home (most pharmacies have information sheets on your prescription medicines; some even offer large-print or Spanish versions).

Do not forget to tell your doctor about all the medicines you are currently taking (not just those for polycystic kidney disease). This includes prescription medicines and the medicines that you buy over the counter. Then your doctor can avoid giving you a new medicine that may not work well with the medications you take now. When talking to your doctor, you may wish to prepare a list of medicines you currently take, the reason you take them, and how you take them. Be sure to include the following information for each:

- Name of medicine

- Reason taken

- Dosage

- Time(s) of day

Also include any over-the-counter medicines, such as:

- Laxatives

- Diet pills

- Vitamins

- Cold medicine

- Aspirin or other pain, headache, or fever medicine

- Cough medicine

- Allergy relief medicine

- Antacids

- Sleeping pills

- Others (include names)

Learning More about Your Medications

Because of historical investments by various organizations and the emergence of the Internet, it has become rather simple to learn about the medications your doctor has recommended for polycystic kidney disease. One such source is the United States Pharmacopeia. In 1820, eleven physicians met in Washington, D.C. to establish the first compendium of standard drugs for the United States. They called this compendium the "U.S. Pharmacopeia (USP)." Today, the USP is a non-profit organization consisting of 800 volunteer scientists, eleven elected officials, and 400 representatives of state associations and colleges of medicine and pharmacy. The USP is located in Rockville, Maryland, and its home page is located at **www.usp.org**. The USP currently provides standards for over 3,700 medications. The resulting USP DI® Advice for the Patient® can be accessed through the National Library of Medicine of the National Institutes of Health. The database is partially derived from lists of federally approved medications in the Food and Drug Administration's (FDA) Drug Approvals database.[40]

While the FDA database is rather large and difficult to navigate, the Phamacopeia is both user-friendly and free to use. It covers more than 9,000 prescription and over-the-counter medications. To access this database, simply type the following hyperlink into your Web browser: **http://www.nlm.nih.gov/medlineplus/druginformation.html**. To view examples of a given medication (brand names, category, description, preparation, proper use, precautions, side effects, etc.), simply follow the hyperlinks indicated within the United States Pharmacopoeia. It is important to read the disclaimer by the United States Pharmacopoeia (**http://www.nlm.nih.gov/medlineplus/drugdisclaimer.html**) before using the information provided.

Of course, we as editors cannot be certain as to what medications you are taking. Therefore, we have compiled a list of medications associated with the treatment of polycystic kidney disease. Once again, due to space limitations, we only list a sample of medications and provide hyperlinks to ample documentation (e.g. typical dosage, side effects, drug-interaction risks, etc.). The following drugs have been mentioned in the Pharmacopeia and other sources as being potentially applicable to polycystic kidney disease:

---

[40] Though cumbersome, the FDA database can be freely browsed at the following site: **www.fda.gov/cder/da/da.htm**.

Ciprofloxacin

- **Ophthalmic - U.S. Brands:** Ciloxan
  http://www.nlm.nih.gov/medlineplus/druginfo/ciprofloxacinop
  hthalmic202655.html

Headache Medicines, Ergot Derivative-Containing

- **Systemic - U.S. Brands:** Cafergot; Cafertine; Cafetrate; D.H.E. 45;
  Ercaf; Ergo-Caff; Ergomar; Ergostat; Gotamine; Migergot; Wigraine
  http://www.nlm.nih.gov/medlineplus/druginfo/headachemedici
  nesergotderivati202216.html

Trimethoprim

- **Systemic - U.S. Brands:** Proloprim; Trimpex
  http://www.nlm.nih.gov/medlineplus/druginfo/trimethoprimsy
  stemic202579.html

Commercial Databases

In addition to the medications listed in the USP above, a number of commercial sites are available by subscription to physicians and their institutions. You may be able to access these sources from your local medical library or your doctor's office.

Reuters Health Drug Database

The Reuters Health Drug Database can be searched by keyword at the hyperlink: **http://www.reutershealth.com/frame2/drug.html**.

Mosby's GenRx

Mosby's GenRx database (also available on CD-Rom and book format) covers 45,000 drug products including generics and international brands. It provides prescribing information, drug interactions, and patient information. Information in Mosby's GenRx database can be obtained at the following hyperlink: **http://www.genrx.com/Mosby/PhyGenRx/group.html**.

Physicians Desk Reference

The Physicians Desk Reference database (also available in CD-Rom and book format) is a full-text drug database. The database is searchable by brand name, generic name or by indication. It features multiple drug interactions reports. Information can be obtained at the following hyperlink: **http://physician.pdr.net/physician/templates/en/acl/psuser_t.htm**.

Other Web Sites

A number of additional Web sites discuss drug information. As an example, you may like to look at **www.drugs.com** which reproduces the information in the Pharmacopeia as well as commercial information. You may also want to consider the Web site of the Medical Letter, Inc. which allows users to download articles on various drugs and therapeutics for a nominal fee: **http://www.medletter.com/**.

Contraindications and Interactions (Hidden Dangers)

Some of the medications mentioned in the previous discussions can be problematic for patients with polycystic kidney disease--not because they are used in the treatment process, but because of contraindications, or side effects. Medications with contraindications are those that could react with drugs used to treat polycystic kidney disease or potentially create deleterious side effects in patients with polycystic kidney disease. You should ask your physician about any contraindications, especially as these might apply to other medications that you may be taking for common ailments.

Drug-drug interactions occur when two or more drugs react with each other. This drug-drug interaction may cause you to experience an unexpected side effect. Drug interactions may make your medications less effective, cause unexpected side effects, or increase the action of a particular drug. Some drug interactions can even be harmful to you.

Be sure to read the label every time you use a nonprescription or prescription drug, and take the time to learn about drug interactions. These precautions may be critical to your health. You can reduce the risk of potentially harmful drug interactions and side effects with a little bit of knowledge and common sense.

Drug labels contain important information about ingredients, uses, warnings, and directions which you should take the time to read and understand. Labels also include warnings about possible drug interactions. Further, drug labels may change as new information becomes available. This is why it's especially important to read the label every time you use a medication. When your doctor prescribes a new drug, discuss all over-the-counter and prescription medications, dietary supplements, vitamins, botanicals, minerals and herbals you take as well as the foods you eat. Ask your pharmacist for the package insert for each prescription drug you take. The package insert provides more information about potential drug interactions.

A Final Warning

At some point, you may hear of alternative medications from friends, relatives, or in the news media. Advertisements may suggest that certain alternative drugs can produce positive results for patients with polycystic kidney disease. Exercise caution--some of these drugs may have fraudulent claims, and others may actually hurt you. The Food and Drug Administration (FDA) is the official U.S. agency charged with discovering which medications are likely to improve the health of patients with polycystic kidney disease. The FDA warns patients to watch out for[41]:

- Secret formulas (real scientists share what they know)

- Amazing breakthroughs or miracle cures (real breakthroughs don't happen very often; when they do, real scientists do not call them amazing or miracles)

- Quick, painless, or guaranteed cures

- If it sounds too good to be true, it probably isn't true.

If you have any questions about any kind of medical treatment, the FDA may have an office near you. Look for their number in the blue pages of the phone book. You can also contact the FDA through its toll-free number, 1-888-INFO-FDA (1-888-463-6332), or on the World Wide Web at **www.fda.gov**.

---

[41] This section has been adapted from **http://www.fda.gov/opacom/lowlit/medfraud.html**

General References

In addition to the resources provided earlier in this chapter, the following general references describe medications (sorted alphabetically by title; hyperlinks provide rankings, information and reviews at Amazon.com):

- **Complete Guide to Prescription and Nonprescription Drugs 2001 (Complete Guide to Prescription and Nonprescription Drugs, 2001)** by H. Winter Griffith, Paperback 16th edition (2001), Medical Surveillance; ISBN: 0942447417;
  http://www.amazon.com/exec/obidos/ASIN/039952634X/icongroupinterna

- **The Essential Guide to Prescription Drugs, 2001** by James J. Rybacki, James W. Long; Paperback - 1274 pages (2001), Harper Resource; ISBN: 0060958162;
  http://www.amazon.com/exec/obidos/ASIN/0060958162/icongroupinterna

- **Handbook of Commonly Prescribed Drugs** by G. John Digregorio, Edward J. Barbieri; Paperback 16th edition (2001), Medical Surveillance; ISBN: 0942447417;
  http://www.amazon.com/exec/obidos/ASIN/0942447417/icongroupinterna

- **Johns Hopkins Complete Home Encyclopedia of Drugs 2nd ed.** by Simeon Margolis (Ed.), Johns Hopkins; Hardcover - 835 pages (2000), Rebus; ISBN: 0929661583;
  http://www.amazon.com/exec/obidos/ASIN/0929661583/icongroupinterna

- **Medical Pocket Reference: Drugs 2002** by Springhouse Paperback 1st edition (2001), Lippincott Williams & Wilkins Publishers; ISBN: 1582550964;
  http://www.amazon.com/exec/obidos/ASIN/1582550964/icongroupinterna

- **PDR** by Medical Economics Staff, Medical Economics Staff Hardcover - 3506 pages 55th edition (2000), Medical Economics Company; ISBN: 1563633752;
  http://www.amazon.com/exec/obidos/ASIN/1563633752/icongroupinterna

- **Pharmacy Simplified: A Glossary of Terms** by James Grogan; Paperback - 432 pages, 1st edition (2001), Delmar Publishers; ISBN: 0766828581;
  http://www.amazon.com/exec/obidos/ASIN/0766828581/icongroupinterna

- **Physician Federal Desk Reference** by Christine B. Fraizer; Paperback 2nd edition (2001), Medicode Inc; ISBN: 1563373971;
  http://www.amazon.com/exec/obidos/ASIN/1563373971/icongroupinterna

- **Physician's Desk Reference Supplements** Paperback - 300 pages, 53 edition (1999), ISBN: 1563632950;
  http://www.amazon.com/exec/obidos/ASIN/1563632950/icongroupinterna

Vocabulary Builder

The following vocabulary builder gives definitions of words used in this chapter that have not been defined in previous chapters:

Ciprofloxacin: A carboxyfluoroquinoline antimicrobial agent that is effective against a wide range of microorganisms. It has been successfully and safely used in the treatment of resistant respiratory, skin, bone, joint, gastrointestinal, urinary, and genital infections. [NIH]

Ophthalmic: Pertaining to the eye. [EU]

APPENDIX B. RESEARCHING ALTERNATIVE MEDICINE

Overview

Complementary and alternative medicine (CAM) is one of the most contentious aspects of modern medical practice. You may have heard of these treatments on the radio or on television. Maybe you have seen articles written about these treatments in magazines, newspapers, or books. Perhaps your friends or doctor have mentioned alternatives.

In this chapter, we will begin by giving you a broad perspective on complementary and alternative therapies. Next, we will introduce you to official information sources on CAM relating to polycystic kidney disease. Finally, at the conclusion of this chapter, we will provide a list of readings on polycystic kidney disease from various authors. We will begin, however, with the National Center for Complementary and Alternative Medicine's (NCCAM) overview of complementary and alternative medicine.

What Is CAM?[42]

Complementary and alternative medicine (CAM) covers a broad range of healing philosophies, approaches, and therapies. Generally, it is defined as those treatments and healthcare practices which are not taught in medical schools, used in hospitals, or reimbursed by medical insurance companies. Many CAM therapies are termed "holistic," which generally means that the healthcare practitioner considers the whole person, including physical, mental, emotional, and spiritual health. Some of these therapies are also known as "preventive," which means that the practitioner educates and

---

[42] Adapted from the NCCAM: **http://nccam.nih.gov/nccam/fcp/faq/index.html#what-is**.

treats the person to prevent health problems from arising, rather than treating symptoms after problems have occurred.

People use CAM treatments and therapies in a variety of ways. Therapies are used alone (often referred to as alternative), in combination with other alternative therapies, or in addition to conventional treatment (sometimes referred to as complementary). Complementary and alternative medicine, or "integrative medicine," includes a broad range of healing philosophies, approaches, and therapies. Some approaches are consistent with physiological principles of Western medicine, while others constitute healing systems with non-Western origins. While some therapies are far outside the realm of accepted Western medical theory and practice, others are becoming established in mainstream medicine.

Complementary and alternative therapies are used in an effort to prevent illness, reduce stress, prevent or reduce side effects and symptoms, or control or cure disease. Some commonly used methods of complementary or alternative therapy include mind/body control interventions such as visualization and relaxation, manual healing including acupressure and massage, homeopathy, vitamins or herbal products, and acupuncture.

What Are the Domains of Alternative Medicine?[43]

The list of CAM practices changes continually. The reason being is that these new practices and therapies are often proved to be safe and effective, and therefore become generally accepted as "mainstream" healthcare practices. Today, CAM practices may be grouped within five major domains: (1) alternative medical systems, (2) mind-body interventions, (3) biologically-based treatments, (4) manipulative and body-based methods, and (5) energy therapies. The individual systems and treatments comprising these categories are too numerous to list in this sourcebook. Thus, only limited examples are provided within each.

Alternative Medical Systems

Alternative medical systems involve complete systems of theory and practice that have evolved independent of, and often prior to, conventional biomedical approaches. Many are traditional systems of medicine that are

---

[43] Adapted from the NCCAM: **http://nccam.nih.gov/nccam/fcp/classify/index.html**

practiced by individual cultures throughout the world, including a number of venerable Asian approaches.

Traditional oriental medicine emphasizes the balance or disturbances of qi (pronounced chi) or vital energy in health and disease, respectively. Traditional oriental medicine consists of a group of techniques and methods including acupuncture, herbal medicine, oriental massage, and qi gong (a form of energy therapy). Acupuncture involves stimulating specific anatomic points in the body for therapeutic purposes, usually by puncturing the skin with a thin needle.

Ayurveda is India's traditional system of medicine. Ayurvedic medicine (meaning "science of life") is a comprehensive system of medicine that places equal emphasis on body, mind, and spirit. Ayurveda strives to restore the innate harmony of the individual. Some of the primary Ayurvedic treatments include diet, exercise, meditation, herbs, massage, exposure to sunlight, and controlled breathing.

Other traditional healing systems have been developed by the world's indigenous populations. These populations include Native American, Aboriginal, African, Middle Eastern, Tibetan, and Central and South American cultures. Homeopathy and naturopathy are also examples of complete alternative medicine systems.

Homeopathic medicine is an unconventional Western system that is based on the principle that "like cures like," i.e., that the same substance that in large doses produces the symptoms of an illness, in very minute doses cures it. Homeopathic health practitioners believe that the more dilute the remedy, the greater its potency. Therefore, they use small doses of specially prepared plant extracts and minerals to stimulate the body's defense mechanisms and healing processes in order to treat illness.

Naturopathic medicine is based on the theory that disease is a manifestation of alterations in the processes by which the body naturally heals itself and emphasizes health restoration rather than disease treatment. Naturopathic physicians employ an array of healing practices, including the following: diet and clinical nutrition, homeopathy, acupuncture, herbal medicine, hydrotherapy (the use of water in a range of temperatures and methods of applications), spinal and soft-tissue manipulation, physical therapies (such as those involving electrical currents, ultrasound, and light), therapeutic counseling, and pharmacology.

Mind-Body Interventions

Mind-body interventions employ a variety of techniques designed to facilitate the mind's capacity to affect bodily function and symptoms. Only a select group of mind-body interventions having well-documented theoretical foundations are considered CAM. For example, patient education and cognitive-behavioral approaches are now considered "mainstream." On the other hand, complementary and alternative medicine includes meditation, certain uses of hypnosis, dance, music, and art therapy, as well as prayer and mental healing.

Biological-Based Therapies

This category of CAM includes natural and biological-based practices, interventions, and products, many of which overlap with conventional medicine's use of dietary supplements. This category includes herbal, special dietary, orthomolecular, and individual biological therapies.

Herbal therapy employs an individual herb or a mixture of herbs for healing purposes. An herb is a plant or plant part that produces and contains chemical substances that act upon the body. Special diet therapies, such as those proposed by Drs. Atkins, Ornish, Pritikin, and Weil, are believed to prevent and/or control illness as well as promote health. Orthomolecular therapies aim to treat disease with varying concentrations of chemicals such as magnesium, melatonin, and mega-doses of vitamins. Biological therapies include, for example, the use of laetrile and shark cartilage to treat cancer and the use of bee pollen to treat autoimmune and inflammatory diseases.

Manipulative and Body-Based Methods

This category includes methods that are based on manipulation and/or movement of the body. For example, chiropractors focus on the relationship between structure and function, primarily pertaining to the spine, and how that relationship affects the preservation and restoration of health. Chiropractors use manipulative therapy as an integral treatment tool.

In contrast, osteopaths place particular emphasis on the musculoskeletal system and practice osteopathic manipulation. Osteopaths believe that all of the body's systems work together and that disturbances in one system may have an impact upon function elsewhere in the body. Massage therapists manipulate the soft tissues of the body to normalize those tissues.

Energy Therapies

Energy therapies focus on energy fields originating within the body (biofields) or those from other sources (electromagnetic fields). Biofield therapies are intended to affect energy fields (the existence of which is not yet experimentally proven) that surround and penetrate the human body. Some forms of energy therapy manipulate biofields by applying pressure and/or manipulating the body by placing the hands in or through these fields. Examples include Qi gong, Reiki and Therapeutic Touch.

Qi gong is a component of traditional oriental medicine that combines movement, meditation, and regulation of breathing to enhance the flow of vital energy (qi) in the body, improve blood circulation, and enhance immune function. Reiki, the Japanese word representing Universal Life Energy, is based on the belief that, by channeling spiritual energy through the practitioner, the spirit is healed and, in turn, heals the physical body. Therapeutic Touch is derived from the ancient technique of "laying-on of hands." It is based on the premises that the therapist's healing force affects the patient's recovery and that healing is promoted when the body's energies are in balance. By passing their hands over the patient, these healers identify energy imbalances.

Bioelectromagnetic-based therapies involve the unconventional use of electromagnetic fields to treat illnesses or manage pain. These therapies are often used to treat asthma, cancer, and migraine headaches. Types of electromagnetic fields which are manipulated in these therapies include pulsed fields, magnetic fields, and alternating current or direct current fields.

Can Alternatives Affect My Treatment?

A critical issue in pursuing complementary alternatives mentioned thus far is the risk that these might have undesirable interactions with your medical treatment. It becomes all the more important to speak with your doctor who can offer advice on the use of alternatives. Official sources confirm this view. Though written for women, we find that the National Women's Health Information Center's advice on pursuing alternative medicine is appropriate for patients of both genders and all ages.[44]

---

[44] Adapted from **http://www.4woman.gov/faq/alternative.htm** .

Is It Okay to Want Both Traditional and Alternative Medicine?

Should you wish to explore non-traditional types of treatment, be sure to discuss all issues concerning treatments and therapies with your healthcare provider, whether a physician or practitioner of complementary and alternative medicine. Competent healthcare management requires knowledge of both conventional and alternative therapies you are taking for the practitioner to have a complete picture of your treatment plan.

The decision to use complementary and alternative treatments is an important one. Consider before selecting an alternative therapy, the safety and effectiveness of the therapy or treatment, the expertise and qualifications of the healthcare practitioner, and the quality of delivery. These topics should be considered when selecting any practitioner or therapy.

Finding CAM References on Polycystic Kidney Disease

Having read the previous discussion, you may be wondering which complementary or alternative treatments might be appropriate for polycystic kidney disease. For the remainder of this chapter, we will direct you to a number of official sources which can assist you in researching studies and publications. Some of these articles are rather technical, so some patience may be required.

National Center for Complementary and Alternative Medicine

The National Center for Complementary and Alternative Medicine (NCCAM) of the National Institutes of Health (**http://nccam.nih.gov**) has created a link to the National Library of Medicine's databases to allow patients to search for articles that specifically relate to polycystic kidney disease and complementary medicine. To search the database, go to the following Web site: **www.nlm.nih.gov/nccam/camonpubmed.html**. Select "CAM on PubMed." Enter "polycystic kidney disease" (or synonyms) into the search box. Click "Go." The following references provide information on particular aspects of complementary and alternative medicine (CAM) that are related to polycystic kidney disease:

- **Conservative long-term treatment of chronic renal failure with keto acid and amino acid supplementation.**
  Author(s): Schmicker R, Vetter K, Lindenau K, Frohling PT, Kokot F.

Source: Infusionsther Klin Ernahr. 1987 October; 14 Suppl 5: 34-8.
http://www.ncbi.nlm.nih.gov:80/entrez/query.fcgi?cmd=Retrieve&db=
PubMed&list_uids=3125108&dopt=Abstract

- **Cures for polycystic kidney diseases?**
  Author(s): Woolf AS.
  Source: Nephrology, Dialysis, Transplantation : Official Publication of the
  European Dialysis and Transplant Association - European Renal
  Association. 1994; 9(10): 1361-2. No Abstract Available.
  http://www.ncbi.nlm.nih.gov:80/entrez/query.fcgi?cmd=Retrieve&db=
  PubMed&list_uids=7816242&dopt=Abstract

- **Diagnostic aspects, functional significance and therapy of simple renal
  cysts. A clinical, radiologic and experimental study.**
  Author(s): Holmberg G.
  Source: Scand J Urol Nephrol Suppl. 1992; 145: 1-48.
  http://www.ncbi.nlm.nih.gov:80/entrez/query.fcgi?cmd=Retrieve&db=
  PubMed&list_uids=1292068&dopt=Abstract

- **Does a low protein diet really slow down the rate of progression of
  chronic renal failure?**
  Author(s): Gretz N, Meisinger E, Strauch M.
  Source: Blood Purification. 1989; 7(1): 33-8. Review.
  http://www.ncbi.nlm.nih.gov:80/entrez/query.fcgi?cmd=Retrieve&db=
  PubMed&list_uids=2645923&dopt=Abstract

- **Dynamics of erythropoiesis following renal transplantation.**
  Author(s): Besarab A, Caro J, Jarrell BE, Francos G, Erslev AJ.
  Source: Kidney International. 1987 October; 32(4): 526-36.
  http://www.ncbi.nlm.nih.gov:80/entrez/query.fcgi?cmd=Retrieve&db=
  PubMed&list_uids=3323595&dopt=Abstract

- **Efficacy of taxol in the orpk mouse model of polycystic kidney disease.**
  Author(s): Sommardahl CS, Woychik RP, Sweeney WE, Avner ED,
  Wilkinson JE.
  Source: Pediatric Nephrology (Berlin, Germany). 1997 December; 11(6):
  728-33.
  http://www.ncbi.nlm.nih.gov:80/entrez/query.fcgi?cmd=Retrieve&db=
  PubMed&list_uids=9438653&dopt=Abstract

- **High dosage metolazone in chronic renal failure.**
  Author(s): Dargie HJ, Allison ME, Kennedy AC, Gray MJ.

Source: British Medical Journal. 1972 October 28; 4(834): 196-8. No Abstract Available.
http://www.ncbi.nlm.nih.gov:80/entrez/query.fcgi?cmd=Retrieve&db=PubMed&list_uids=5082545&dopt=Abstract

- **In vitro formation of cysts derived from a rat model of autosomal dominant polycystic kidney disease.**
  Author(s): Pey R, Hafner M, Schieren G, Bach J, Gretz N.
  Source: Nephrology, Dialysis, Transplantation : Official Publication of the European Dialysis and Transplant Association - European Renal Association. 1996; 11 Suppl 6: 58-61. Review.
  http://www.ncbi.nlm.nih.gov:80/entrez/query.fcgi?cmd=Retrieve&db=PubMed&list_uids=9044330&dopt=Abstract

- **Infusion of total dose iron versus oral iron supplementation in ambulatory peritoneal dialysis patients: a prospective, cross-over trial.**
  Author(s): Ahsan N.
  Source: Adv Perit Dial. 2000; 16: 80-4.
  http://www.ncbi.nlm.nih.gov:80/entrez/query.fcgi?cmd=Retrieve&db=PubMed&list_uids=11045266&dopt=Abstract

- **Initial effect of enalapril on kidney function in patients with moderate to severe chronic nephropathy.**
  Author(s): Kamper AL, Thomsen HS, Nielsen SL, Strandgaard S.
  Source: Scandinavian Journal of Urology and Nephrology. 1990; 24(1): 69-73.
  http://www.ncbi.nlm.nih.gov:80/entrez/query.fcgi?cmd=Retrieve&db=PubMed&list_uids=2157277&dopt=Abstract

- **Massive bilateral nephroblastomatosis in a 13-year-old-girl.**
  Author(s): Pichler E, Jurgenssen OA, Balzar E, Pinggera WF, Wolf A, Wagner O, Reinartz G, Czembirek H, Syre G.
  Source: European Journal of Pediatrics. 1982 May; 138(3): 231-6. No Abstract Available.
  http://www.ncbi.nlm.nih.gov:80/entrez/query.fcgi?cmd=Retrieve&db=PubMed&list_uids=6288384&dopt=Abstract

- **Matrix metalloproteinases and TIMPS in cultured C57BL/6J-cpk kidney tubules.**
  Author(s): Rankin CA, Suzuki K, Itoh Y, Ziemer DM, Grantham JJ, Calvet JP, Nagase H.

Source: Kidney International. 1996 September; 50(3): 835-44.
http://www.ncbi.nlm.nih.gov:80/entrez/query.fcgi?cmd=Retrieve&db=
PubMed&list_uids=8872958&dopt=Abstract

- **Microtubule active taxanes inhibit polycystic kidney disease progression in cpk mice.**
  Author(s): Woo DD, Tabancay AP Jr, Wang CJ.
  Source: Kidney International. 1997 May; 51(5): 1613-8.
  http://www.ncbi.nlm.nih.gov:80/entrez/query.fcgi?cmd=Retrieve&db=
  PubMed&list_uids=9150481&dopt=Abstract

- **Modification of polycystic kidney disease and fatty acid status by soy protein diet.**
  Author(s): Ogborn MR, Nitschmann E, Weiler HA, Bankovic-Calic N.
  Source: Kidney International. 2000 January; 57(1): 159-66.
  http://www.ncbi.nlm.nih.gov:80/entrez/query.fcgi?cmd=Retrieve&db=
  PubMed&list_uids=10620197&dopt=Abstract

- **Observations in a Saudi-Arabian dialysis population over a 13-year period.**
  Author(s): Hussein MM, Mooij JM, Roujouleh H, el-Sayed H.
  Source: Nephrology, Dialysis, Transplantation : Official Publication of the European Dialysis and Transplant Association - European Renal Association. 1994; 9(8): 1072-6.
  http://www.ncbi.nlm.nih.gov:80/entrez/query.fcgi?cmd=Retrieve&db=
  PubMed&list_uids=7800203&dopt=Abstract

- **Pain management in polycystic kidney disease.**
  Author(s): Bajwa ZH, Gupta S, Warfield CA, Steinman TI.
  Source: Kidney International. 2001 November; 60(5): 1631-44. Review.
  http://www.ncbi.nlm.nih.gov:80/entrez/query.fcgi?cmd=Retrieve&db=
  PubMed&list_uids=11703580&dopt=Abstract

- **Predictors of renal function in diabetic and non-diabetic renal disease.**
  Author(s): Feehally J, Taverner D, Burden AC, Walls J.
  Source: Clinica Chimica Acta; International Journal of Clinical Chemistry. 1983 September 30; 133(2): 169-75.
  http://www.ncbi.nlm.nih.gov:80/entrez/query.fcgi?cmd=Retrieve&db=
  PubMed&list_uids=6354517&dopt=Abstract

- **Racial origin and primary renal diagnosis in 771 patients with end-stage renal disease.**
  Author(s): Pazianas M, Eastwood JB, MacRae KD, Phillips ME.
  Source: Nephrology, Dialysis, Transplantation : Official Publication of the European Dialysis and Transplant Association - European Renal Association. 1991; 6(12): 931-5.
  http://www.ncbi.nlm.nih.gov:80/entrez/query.fcgi?cmd=Retrieve&db=PubMed&list_uids=1798591&dopt=Abstract

- **Rate of functional deterioration in polycystic kidney disease.**
  Author(s): Franz KA, Reubi FC.
  Source: Kidney International. 1983 March; 23(3): 526-9.
  http://www.ncbi.nlm.nih.gov:80/entrez/query.fcgi?cmd=Retrieve&db=PubMed&list_uids=6405076&dopt=Abstract

- **Serum levels of the soluble interleukin-2 receptor are dependent on the kidney function.**
  Author(s): Nassberger L, Sturfelt G, Thysell H.
  Source: American Journal of Nephrology. 1992; 12(6): 401-5.
  http://www.ncbi.nlm.nih.gov:80/entrez/query.fcgi?cmd=Retrieve&db=PubMed&list_uids=1292338&dopt=Abstract

- **Tamm-Horsfall protein antibody in patients with end-stage kidney disease.**
  Author(s): Work J, Andriole VT.
  Source: Yale J Biol Med. 1980 March-April; 53(2): 133-48.
  http://www.ncbi.nlm.nih.gov:80/entrez/query.fcgi?cmd=Retrieve&db=PubMed&list_uids=7395272&dopt=Abstract

- **Taxol inhibits progression of congenital polycystic kidney disease.**
  Author(s): Woo DD, Miao SY, Pelayo JC, Woolf AS.
  Source: Nature. 1994 April 21; 368(6473): 750-3.
  http://www.ncbi.nlm.nih.gov:80/entrez/query.fcgi?cmd=Retrieve&db=PubMed&list_uids=7908721&dopt=Abstract

- **The effect of dietary flaxseed supplementation on organic anion and osmolyte content and excretion in rat polycystic kidney disease.**
  Author(s): Ogborn MR, Nitschmann E, Bankovic-Calic N, Buist R, Peeling J.

Source: Biochemistry and Cell Biology = Biochimie Et Biologie Cellulaire. 1998; 76(2-3): 553-9.
http://www.ncbi.nlm.nih.gov:80/entrez/query.fcgi?cmd=Retrieve&db=PubMed&list_uids=9923725&dopt=Abstract

- **The effect of paclitaxel on the progression of polycystic kidney disease in rodents.**
Author(s): Martinez JR, Cowley BD, Gattone VH 2nd, Nagao S, Yamaguchi T, Kaneta S, Takahashi H, Grantham JJ.
Source: American Journal of Kidney Diseases : the Official Journal of the National Kidney Foundation. 1997 March; 29(3): 435-44.
http://www.ncbi.nlm.nih.gov:80/entrez/query.fcgi?cmd=Retrieve&db=PubMed&list_uids=9041221&dopt=Abstract

- **The maximal tubular reabsorption of phosphate in relation to serum parathyroid hormone.**
Author(s): Madsen S, Olgaard K, Ladefoged J.
Source: Advances in Experimental Medicine and Biology. 1977; 81: 141-8.
http://www.ncbi.nlm.nih.gov:80/entrez/query.fcgi?cmd=Retrieve&db=PubMed&list_uids=899923&dopt=Abstract

- **The molecular and structural basis of hearing impairment in mice with the cpk mutant gene.**
Author(s): Cho H, Buchanan J, Strong D, Yamada Y, Yoo TJ.
Source: Annals of the New York Academy of Sciences. 1991; 630: 262-4.
http://www.ncbi.nlm.nih.gov:80/entrez/query.fcgi?cmd=Retrieve&db=PubMed&list_uids=1952600&dopt=Abstract

Additional Web Resources

A number of additional Web sites offer encyclopedic information covering CAM and related topics. The following is a representative sample:

- Alternative Medicine Foundation, Inc.: **http://www.herbmed.org/**
- AOL: **http://search.aol.com/cat.adp?id=169&layer=&from=subcats**
- Chinese Medicine: **http://www.newcenturynutrition.com/**
- drkoop.com®: **http://www.drkoop.com/InteractiveMedicine/IndexC.html**
- Family Village: **http://www.familyvillage.wisc.edu/med_altn.htm**

- Google: **http://directory.google.com/Top/Health/Alternative/**

- Healthnotes: **http://www.thedacare.org/healthnotes/**

- Open Directory Project: **http://dmoz.org/Health/Alternative/**

- TPN.com: **http://www.tnp.com/**

- Yahoo.com: **http://dir.yahoo.com/Health/Alternative_Medicine/**

- WebMD®Health: **http://my.webmd.com/drugs_and_herbs**

- WellNet: **http://www.wellnet.ca/herbsa-c.htm**

- WholeHealthMD.com: **http://www.wholehealthmd.com/reflib/0,1529,,00.html**

General References

A good place to find general background information on CAM is the National Library of Medicine. It has prepared within the MEDLINEplus system an information topic page dedicated to complementary and alternative medicine. To access this page, go to the MEDLINEplus site at: **www.nlm.nih.gov/medlineplus/alternativemedicine.html.** This Web site provides a general overview of various topics and can lead to a number of general sources. The following additional references describe, in broad terms, alternative and complementary medicine (sorted alphabetically by title; hyperlinks provide rankings, information, and reviews at Amazon.com):

- **Alternative Medicine for Dummies** by James Dillard (Author); Audio Cassette, Abridged edition (1998), Harper Audio; ISBN: 0694520659; **http://www.amazon.com/exec/obidos/ASIN/0694520659/icongroupinterna**

- **Complementary and Alternative Medicine Secrets** by W. Kohatsu (Editor); Hardcover (2001), Hanley & Belfus; ISBN: 1560534400; **http://www.amazon.com/exec/obidos/ASIN/1560534400/icongroupinterna**

- **Dictionary of Alternative Medicine** by J. C. Segen; Paperback-2nd edition (2001), Appleton & Lange; ISBN: 0838516211; **http://www.amazon.com/exec/obidos/ASIN/0838516211/icongroupinterna**

- **Eat, Drink, and Be Healthy: The Harvard Medical School Guide to Healthy Eating** by Walter C. Willett, MD, et al; Hardcover - 352 pages (2001), Simon & Schuster; ISBN: 0684863375; **http://www.amazon.com/exec/obidos/ASIN/0684863375/icongroupinterna**

- **Encyclopedia of Natural Medicine, Revised 2nd Edition** by Michael T. Murray, Joseph E. Pizzorno; Paperback - 960 pages, 2nd Rev edition (1997),

Prima Publishing; ISBN: 0761511571;
http://www.amazon.com/exec/obidos/ASIN/0761511571/icongroupinterna

- **Herbs for the Urinary Tract: Herbal Relief for Kidney Stones, Bladder Infections and Other Problems of the Urinary Tract** by Michael Moore; Paperback - 96 pages (June 1998), McGraw Hill - NTC; ISBN: 0879838159; http://www.amazon.com/exec/obidos/ASIN/0879838159/icongroupinterna

- **Integrative Medicine: An Introduction to the Art & Science of Healing** by Andrew Weil (Author); Audio Cassette, Unabridged edition (2001), Sounds True; ISBN: 1564558541; http://www.amazon.com/exec/obidos/ASIN/1564558541/icongroupinterna

- **New Encyclopedia of Herbs & Their Uses** by Deni Bown; Hardcover - 448 pages, Revised edition (2001), DK Publishing; ISBN: 078948031X; http://www.amazon.com/exec/obidos/ASIN/078948031X/icongroupinterna

- **Textbook of Complementary and Alternative Medicine** by Wayne B. Jonas; Hardcover (2003), Lippincott, Williams & Wilkins; ISBN: 0683044370; http://www.amazon.com/exec/obidos/ASIN/0683044370/icongroupinterna

For additional information on complementary and alternative medicine, ask your doctor or write to:

National Institutes of Health
National Center for Complementary and Alternative Medicine Clearinghouse
P. O. Box 8218
Silver Spring, MD 20907-8218

Vocabulary Builder

The following vocabulary builder gives definitions of words used in this chapter that have not been defined in previous chapters:

Antibody: An immunoglobulin molecule that has a specific amino acid sequence by virtue of which it interacts only with the antigen that induced its synthesis in cells of the lymphoid series (especially plasma cells), or with antigen closely related to it. Antibodies are classified according to their ode of action as agglutinins, bacteriolysins, haemolysins, opsonins, precipitins, etc. [EU]

Enalapril: An angiotensin-converting enzyme inhibitor that is used to treat hypertension. [NIH]

Metolazone: A potent, long acting diuretic useful in chronic renal disease. It also tends to lower blood pressure and increase potassium loss. [NIH]

Parathyroid: 1. situated beside the thyroid gland. 2. one of the parathyroid glands. 3. a sterile preparation of the water-soluble principle(s) of the parathyroid glands, ad-ministered parenterally as an antihypocalcaemic, especially in the treatment of acute hypoparathyroidism with tetany. [EU]

Reabsorption: 1. the act or process of absorbing again, as the selective absorption by the kidneys of substances (glucose, proteins, sodium, etc.) already secreted into the renal tubules, and their return to the circulating blood. 2. resorption. [EU]

APPENDIX C. RESEARCHING NUTRITION

Overview

Since the time of Hippocrates, doctors have understood the importance of diet and nutrition to patients' health and well-being. Since then, they have accumulated an impressive archive of studies and knowledge dedicated to this subject. Based on their experience, doctors and healthcare providers may recommend particular dietary supplements to patients with polycystic kidney disease. Any dietary recommendation is based on a patient's age, body mass, gender, lifestyle, eating habits, food preferences, and health condition. It is therefore likely that different patients with polycystic kidney disease may be given different recommendations. Some recommendations may be directly related to polycystic kidney disease, while others may be more related to the patient's general health. These recommendations, themselves, may differ from what official sources recommend for the average person.

In this chapter we will begin by briefly reviewing the essentials of diet and nutrition that will broadly frame more detailed discussions of polycystic kidney disease. We will then show you how to find studies dedicated specifically to nutrition and polycystic kidney disease.

Food and Nutrition: General Principles

What Are Essential Foods?

Food is generally viewed by official sources as consisting of six basic elements: (1) fluids, (2) carbohydrates, (3) protein, (4) fats, (5) vitamins, and

(6) minerals. Consuming a combination of these elements is considered to be a healthy diet:

- **Fluids** are essential to human life as 80-percent of the body is composed of water. Water is lost via urination, sweating, diarrhea, vomiting, diuretics (drugs that increase urination), caffeine, and physical exertion.

- **Carbohydrates** are the main source for human energy (thermoregulation) and the bulk of typical diets. They are mostly classified as being either simple or complex. Simple carbohydrates include sugars which are often consumed in the form of cookies, candies, or cakes. Complex carbohydrates consist of starches and dietary fibers. Starches are consumed in the form of pastas, breads, potatoes, rice, and other foods. Soluble fibers can be eaten in the form of certain vegetables, fruits, oats, and legumes. Insoluble fibers include brown rice, whole grains, certain fruits, wheat bran and legumes.

- **Proteins** are eaten to build and repair human tissues. Some foods that are high in protein are also high in fat and calories. Food sources for protein include nuts, meat, fish, cheese, and other dairy products.

- **Fats** are consumed for both energy and the absorption of certain vitamins. There are many types of fats, with many general publications recommending the intake of unsaturated fats or those low in cholesterol.

Vitamins and minerals are fundamental to human health, growth, and, in some cases, disease prevention. Most are consumed in your diet (exceptions being vitamins K and D which are produced by intestinal bacteria and sunlight on the skin, respectively). Each vitamin and mineral plays a different role in health. The following outlines essential vitamins:

- **Vitamin A** is important to the health of your eyes, hair, bones, and skin; sources of vitamin A include foods such as eggs, carrots, and cantaloupe.

- **Vitamin B^1**, also known as thiamine, is important for your nervous system and energy production; food sources for thiamine include meat, peas, fortified cereals, bread, and whole grains.

- **Vitamin B^2**, also known as riboflavin, is important for your nervous system and muscles, but is also involved in the release of proteins from nutrients; food sources for riboflavin include dairy products, leafy vegetables, meat, and eggs.

- **Vitamin B^3**, also known as niacin, is important for healthy skin and helps the body use energy; food sources for niacin include peas, peanuts, fish, and whole grains

- **Vitamin B^6**, also known as pyridoxine, is important for the regulation of cells in the nervous system and is vital for blood formation; food sources for pyridoxine include bananas, whole grains, meat, and fish.

- **Vitamin B^{12}** is vital for a healthy nervous system and for the growth of red blood cells in bone marrow; food sources for vitamin B^{12} include yeast, milk, fish, eggs, and meat.

- **Vitamin C** allows the body's immune system to fight various diseases, strengthens body tissue, and improves the body's use of iron; food sources for vitamin C include a wide variety of fruits and vegetables.

- **Vitamin D** helps the body absorb calcium which strengthens bones and teeth; food sources for vitamin D include oily fish and dairy products.

- **Vitamin E** can help protect certain organs and tissues from various degenerative diseases; food sources for vitamin E include margarine, vegetables, eggs, and fish.

- **Vitamin K** is essential for bone formation and blood clotting; common food sources for vitamin K include leafy green vegetables.

- **Folic Acid** maintains healthy cells and blood and, when taken by a pregnant woman, can prevent her fetus from developing neural tube defects; food sources for folic acid include nuts, fortified breads, leafy green vegetables, and whole grains.

It should be noted that one can overdose on certain vitamins which become toxic if consumed in excess (e.g. vitamin A, D, E and K).

Like vitamins, minerals are chemicals that are required by the body to remain in good health. Because the human body does not manufacture these chemicals internally, we obtain them from food and other dietary sources. The more important minerals include:

- **Calcium** is needed for healthy bones, teeth, and muscles, but also helps the nervous system function; food sources for calcium include dry beans, peas, eggs, and dairy products.

- **Chromium** is helpful in regulating sugar levels in blood; food sources for chromium include egg yolks, raw sugar, cheese, nuts, beets, whole grains, and meat.

- **Fluoride** is used by the body to help prevent tooth decay and to reinforce bone strength; sources of fluoride include drinking water and certain brands of toothpaste.

- **Iodine** helps regulate the body's use of energy by synthesizing into the hormone thyroxine; food sources include leafy green vegetables, nuts, egg yolks, and red meat.

- **Iron** helps maintain muscles and the formation of red blood cells and certain proteins; food sources for iron include meat, dairy products, eggs, and leafy green vegetables.

- **Magnesium** is important for the production of DNA, as well as for healthy teeth, bones, muscles, and nerves; food sources for magnesium include dried fruit, dark green vegetables, nuts, and seafood.

- **Phosphorous** is used by the body to work with calcium to form bones and teeth; food sources for phosphorous include eggs, meat, cereals, and dairy products.

- **Selenium** primarily helps maintain normal heart and liver functions; food sources for selenium include wholegrain cereals, fish, meat, and dairy products.

- **Zinc** helps wounds heal, the formation of sperm, and encourage rapid growth and energy; food sources include dried beans, shellfish, eggs, and nuts.

The United States government periodically publishes recommended diets and consumption levels of the various elements of food. Again, your doctor may encourage deviations from the average official recommendation based on your specific condition. To learn more about basic dietary guidelines, visit the Web site: **http://www.health.gov/dietaryguidelines/**. Based on these guidelines, many foods are required to list the nutrition levels on the food's packaging. Labeling Requirements are listed at the following site maintained by the Food and Drug Administration: **http://www.cfsan.fda.gov/~dms/lab-cons.html**. When interpreting these requirements, the government recommends that consumers become familiar with the following abbreviations before reading FDA literature:[45]

- **DVs (Daily Values):** A new dietary reference term that will appear on the food label. It is made up of two sets of references, DRVs and RDIs.

- **DRVs (Daily Reference Values):** A set of dietary references that applies to fat, saturated fat, cholesterol, carbohydrate, protein, fiber, sodium, and potassium.

- **RDIs (Reference Daily Intakes):** A set of dietary references based on the Recommended Dietary Allowances for essential vitamins and minerals

---

[45] Adapted from the FDA: **http://www.fda.gov/fdac/special/foodlabel/dvs.html**.

and, in selected groups, protein. The name "RDI" replaces the term "U.S. RDA."

- **RDAs (Recommended Dietary Allowances):** A set of estimated nutrient allowances established by the National Academy of Sciences. It is updated periodically to reflect current scientific knowledge.

What Are Dietary Supplements?[46]

Dietary supplements are widely available through many commercial sources, including health food stores, grocery stores, pharmacies, and by mail. Dietary supplements are provided in many forms including tablets, capsules, powders, gel-tabs, extracts, and liquids. Historically in the United States, the most prevalent type of dietary supplement was a multivitamin/mineral tablet or capsule that was available in pharmacies, either by prescription or "over the counter." Supplements containing strictly herbal preparations were less widely available. Currently in the United States, a wide array of supplement products are available, including vitamin, mineral, other nutrients, and botanical supplements as well as ingredients and extracts of animal and plant origin.

The Office of Dietary Supplements (ODS) of the National Institutes of Health is the official agency of the United States which has the expressed goal of acquiring "new knowledge to help prevent, detect, diagnose, and treat disease and disability, from the rarest genetic disorder to the common cold."[47] According to the ODS, dietary supplements can have an important impact on the prevention and management of disease and on the maintenance of health.[48] The ODS notes that considerable research on the effects of dietary supplements has been conducted in Asia and Europe where the use of plant products, in particular, has a long tradition. However, the overwhelming majority of supplements have not been studied scientifically.

---

[46] This discussion has been adapted from the NIH: **http://ods.od.nih.gov/whatare/whatare.html**.

[47] Contact: The Office of Dietary Supplements, National Institutes of Health, Building 31, Room 1B29, 31 Center Drive, MSC 2086, Bethesda, Maryland 20892-2086, Tel: (301) 435-2920, Fax: (301) 480-1845, E-mail: **ods@nih.gov**.

[48] Adapted from **http://ods.od.nih.gov/about/about.html**. The Dietary Supplement Health and Education Act defines dietary supplements as "a product (other than tobacco) intended to supplement the diet that bears or contains one or more of the following dietary ingredients: a vitamin, mineral, amino acid, herb or other botanical; or a dietary substance for use to supplement the diet by increasing the total dietary intake; or a concentrate, metabolite, constituent, extract, or combination of any ingredient described above; and intended for ingestion in the form of a capsule, powder, softgel, or gelcap, and not represented as a conventional food or as a sole item of a meal or the diet."

To explore the role of dietary supplements in the improvement of health care, the ODS plans, organizes, and supports conferences, workshops, and symposia on scientific topics related to dietary supplements. The ODS often works in conjunction with other NIH Institutes and Centers, other government agencies, professional organizations, and public advocacy groups.

To learn more about official information on dietary supplements, visit the ODS site at **http://ods.od.nih.gov/whatare/whatare.html**. Or contact:

> The Office of Dietary Supplements
> National Institutes of Health
> Building 31, Room 1B29
> 31 Center Drive, MSC 2086
> Bethesda, Maryland 20892-2086
> Tel: (301) 435-2920
> Fax: (301) 480-1845
> E-mail: ods@nih.gov

Finding Studies on Polycystic Kidney Disease

The NIH maintains an office dedicated to patient nutrition and diet. The National Institutes of Health's Office of Dietary Supplements (ODS) offers a searchable bibliographic database called the IBIDS (International Bibliographic Information on Dietary Supplements). The IBIDS contains over 460,000 scientific citations and summaries about dietary supplements and nutrition as well as references to published international, scientific literature on dietary supplements such as vitamins, minerals, and botanicals.[49] IBIDS is available to the public free of charge through the ODS Internet page: **http://ods.od.nih.gov/databases/ibids.html**.

After entering the search area, you have three choices: (1) IBIDS Consumer Database, (2) Full IBIDS Database, or (3) Peer Reviewed Citations Only. We recommend that you start with the Consumer Database. While you may not find references for the topics that are of most interest to you, check back periodically as this database is frequently updated. More studies can be found by searching the Full IBIDS Database. Healthcare professionals and

---

[49] Adapted from **http://ods.od.nih.gov**. IBIDS is produced by the Office of Dietary Supplements (ODS) at he National Institutes of Health to assist the public, healthcare providers, educators, and researchers in locating credible, scientific information on dietary supplements. IBIDS was developed and will be maintained through an interagency partnership with the Food and Nutrition Information Center of the National Agricultural Library, U.S. Department of Agriculture.

researchers generally use the third option, which lists peer-reviewed citations. In all cases, we suggest that you take advantage of the "Advanced Search" option that allows you to retrieve up to 100 fully explained references in a comprehensive format. Type "polycystic kidney disease" (or synonyms) into the search box. To narrow the search, you can also select the "Title" field.

The following information is typical of that found when using the "Full IBIDS Database" when searching using "polycystic kidney disease" (or a synonym):

- **Abnormal lipid and fatty acid compositions of kidneys from mice with polycystic kidney disease.**
  Author(s): University of Guelph, Department of Nutritional Sciences, Ontario, Canada.
  Source: Aukema, H M Yamaguchi, T Takahashi, H Celi, B Holub, B J Lipids. 1992 June; 27(6): 429-35 0024-4201

- **Basement membrane chondroitin sulfate proteoglycan alterations in a rat model of polycystic kidney disease.**
  Author(s): Department of Cell Biology, University of Alabama at Birmingham 35294-0019.
  Source: Ehara, T Carone, F A McCarthy, K J Couchman, J R Am-J-Pathol. 1994 March; 144(3): 612-21 0002-9440

- **Borderline hypertensive autosomal dominant polycystic kidney disease patients have enhanced production of renal dopamine. Normalization of renal haemodynamics by DOPA infusion.**
  Author(s): Department of Nephrology, University Hospital Leiden, The Netherlands.
  Source: Barendregt, J N Florijn, K W Muizert, Y Chang, P C Nephrol-Dial-Transplant. 1995; 10(8): 1332-41 0931-0509

- **Cellular activation triggered by the autosomal dominant polycystic kidney disease gene product PKD2.**
  Author(s): Department of Medicine, Renal Division Beth Israel Deaconess Medical Center, Boston, Massachusetts 02215, USA.
  Source: Arnould, T Sellin, L Benzing, T Tsiokas, L Cohen, H T Kim, E Walz, G Mol-Cell-Biol. 1999 May; 19(5): 3423-34 0270-7306

- **Chlamydomonas IFT88 and its mouse homologue, polycystic kidney disease gene Tg737, are required for assembly of cilia and flagella.**
  Source: Pazour, G.J. Dickert, B.L. Vucica, Y. Seeley, E.S. Rosenbaum, J.L. Witman, G.B. Cole, D.G. J-cell-biol. New York : Rockefeller University Press, 1962-. October 30, 2000. volume 151 (3) page 709-718. 0021-9525

- **Chronic caffeine consumption exacerbates hypertension in rats with polycystic kidney disease.**
  Author(s): Department of Cellular and Integrative Physiology, Indiana University School of Medicine, Indianapolis, IN 46202, USA. gtanner@iupui.edu
  Source: Tanner, G A Tanner, J A Am-J-Kidney-Dis. 2001 November; 38(5): 1089-95 1523-6838

- **Dietary betaine modifies hepatic metabolism but not renal injury in rat polycystic kidney disease.**
  Author(s): Department of Pediatrics and Child Health, University of Manitoba, Winnipeg, Manitoba, Canada R3A 1S1. mogborn@hsc.mb.ca
  Source: Ogborn, M R Nitschmann, E Bankovic Calic, N Buist, R Peeling, J Am-J-Physiol-Gastrointest-Liver-Physiol. 2000 December; 279(6): G1162-8 0193-1857

- **Dietary soy protein effects on inherited polycystic kidney disease are influenced by gender and protein level.**
  Author(s): Department of Nutrition and Food Sciences, and Center for Research on Women's Health, Texas Woman's University, Denton 76204-5888, USA. haukema@twu.edu
  Source: Aukema, H M Housini, I Rawling, J M J-Am-Soc-Nephrol. 1999 February; 10(2): 300-8 1046-6673

- **Differences in hormonal and renal vascular responses between normotensive patients with autosomal dominant polycystic kidney disease and unaffected family members.**
  Author(s): Department of Medicine, Memorial University of Newfoundland, St. John's, Canada.
  Source: Barrett, B J Foley, R Morgan, J Hefferton, D Parfrey, P Kidney-Int. 1994 October; 46(4): 1118-23 0085-2538

- **Diphenylthiazole-induced changes in renal ultrastructure and enzymology: toxicologic mechanisms in polycystic kidney disease?**
  Author(s): University of Illinois College of Medicine, Peoria.
  Source: Hjelle, J T Hjelle, J J Maziasz, T J Carone, F A J-Pharmacol-Exp-Ther. 1987 November; 243(2): 758-66 0022-3565

- **Effect of a low-protein diet on the rate of progression of chronic renal failure in patients with polycystic kidney disease.**
  Author(s): Clinic of Nephrology, Klinikum Mannheim, University of Heidelberg, FRG.
  Source: Gretz, N Strauch, M Contrib-Nephrol. 1992; 9793-100 0302-5144

- **Effect of dietary soy protein and genistein on disease progression in mice with polycystic kidney disease.**
  Author(s): Department of Human Biology and Nutritional Sciences, University of Guelph, Ontario, Canada.
  Source: Tomobe, K Philbrick, D J Ogborn, M R Takahashi, H Holub, B J Am-J-Kidney-Dis. 1998 January; 31(1): 55-61 0272-6386

- **Effect of probucol in a murine model of slowly progressive polycystic kidney disease.**
  Author(s): Institute for Comprehensive Medical Science and the Department of Pathology, School of Medicine, Fujita Health University, Toyoake, Japan.
  Source: Nagao, S Yamaguchi, T Kasahara, M Kusaka, M Matsuda, J Ogiso, N Takahashi, H Grantham, J J Am-J-Kidney-Dis. 2000 February; 35(2): 221-6 0272-6386

- **Effect of sodium chloride, enalapril, and losartan on the development of polycystic kidney disease in Han:SPRD rats.**
  Author(s): Department of Pediatrics, Mayo Clinic, Rochester, MN 55905.
  Source: Keith, D S Torres, V E Johnson, C M Holley, K E Am-J-Kidney-Dis. 1994 September; 24(3): 491-8 0272-6386

- **Effects of dietary fish oil on survival and renal fatty acid composition in murine polycystic kidney disease.**
  Source: Aukema, H.M. Yamaguchi, T. Takahashi, H. Philbrick, D.J. Holub, B.J. Nutr-Res. Tarrytown, N.Y. : Pergamon Press. November 1992. volume 12 (11) page 1383-1392. 0271-5317

- **Effects of dietary protein restriction and oil type on the early progression of murine polycystic kidney disease.**
  Author(s): Department of Nutritional Sciences, University of Guelph, Ontario, Canada.
  Source: Aukema, H M Ogborn, M R Tomobe, K Takahashi, H Hibino, T Holub, B J Kidney-Int. 1992 October; 42(4): 837-42 0085-2538

- **Effects of dietary supplementation with n-3 fatty acids on kidney morphology and the fatty acid composition of phospholipids and triglycerides from mice with polycystic kidney disease.**
  Author(s): Department of Nutritional Sciences, University of Guelph, Ontario, Canada.
  Source: Yamaguchi, T Valli, V E Philbrick, D Holub, B Yoshida, K Takahashi, H Res-Commun-Chem-Pathol-Pharmacol. 1990 September; 69(3): 335-51 0034-5164

- **Effects of lithium chloride and ethacrynic acid on experimental polycystic kidney disease.**
  Author(s): Department of Pediatrics, Dalhousie University, Halifax, Nova Scotia.
  Source: Crocker, J F McDonald, A T Clin-Invest-Med. 1988 February; 11(1): 16-21 0147-958X

- **Effects of potassium citrate/citric acid intake in a mouse model of polycystic kidney disease.**
  Author(s): Department of Physiology and Biophysics, Indiana University School of Medicine, Indianapolis, IN 46202, USA. gtanner@iupui.edu
  Source: Tanner, G A Vijayalakshmi, K Tanner, J A Nephron. 2000 March; 84(3): 270-3 0028-2766

- **Endothelium-dependent relaxation of small resistance vessels is impaired in patients with autosomal dominant polycystic kidney disease.**
  Author(s): Departments of Nephrology and Medicine, Herlev Hospital, Denmark. wangdan9090@hotmail.com
  Source: Wang, D Iversen, J Strandgaard, S J-Am-Soc-Nephrol. 2000 August; 11(8): 1371-6 1046-6673

Federal Resources on Nutrition

In addition to the IBIDS, the United States Department of Health and Human Services (HHS) and the United States Department of Agriculture (USDA) provide many sources of information on general nutrition and health. Recommended resources include:

- healthfinder®, HHS's gateway to health information, including diet and nutrition:
  http://www.healthfinder.gov/scripts/SearchContext.asp?topic=238&page=0

- The United States Department of Agriculture's Web site dedicated to nutrition information: **www.nutrition.gov**

- The Food and Drug Administration's Web site for federal food safety information: **www.foodsafety.gov**

- The National Action Plan on Overweight and Obesity sponsored by the United States Surgeon General:
  http://www.surgeongeneral.gov/topics/obesity/

- The Center for Food Safety and Applied Nutrition has an Internet site sponsored by the Food and Drug Administration and the Department of Health and Human Services: **http://vm.cfsan.fda.gov/**

- Center for Nutrition Policy and Promotion sponsored by the United States Department of Agriculture: **http://www.usda.gov/cnpp/**

- Food and Nutrition Information Center, National Agricultural Library sponsored by the United States Department of Agriculture: **http://www.nal.usda.gov/fnic/**

- Food and Nutrition Service sponsored by the United States Department of Agriculture: **http://www.fns.usda.gov/fns/**

Additional Web Resources

A number of additional Web sites offer encyclopedic information covering food and nutrition. The following is a representative sample:

- AOL: **http://search.aol.com/cat.adp?id=174&layer=&from=subcats**

- Family Village: **http://www.familyvillage.wisc.edu/med_nutrition.html**

- Google: **http://directory.google.com/Top/Health/Nutrition/**

- Healthnotes: **http://www.thedacare.org/healthnotes/**

- Open Directory Project: **http://dmoz.org/Health/Nutrition/**

- Yahoo.com: **http://dir.yahoo.com/Health/Nutrition/**

- WebMD®Health: **http://my.webmd.com/nutrition**

- WholeHealthMD.com: **http://www.wholehealthmd.com/reflib/0,1529,,00.html**

Vocabulary Builder

The following vocabulary builder defines words used in the references in this chapter that have not been defined in previous chapters:

Bacteria: Unicellular prokaryotic microorganisms which generally possess rigid cell walls, multiply by cell division, and exhibit three principal forms: round or coccal, rodlike or bacillary, and spiral or spirochetal. [NIH]

Capsules: Hard or soft soluble containers used for the oral administration of medicine. [NIH]

Cholesterol: The principal sterol of all higher animals, distributed in body tissues, especially the brain and spinal cord, and in animal fats and oils. [NIH]

Degenerative: Undergoing degeneration : tending to degenerate; having the character of or involving degeneration; causing or tending to cause degeneration. [EU]

Diarrhea: Passage of excessively liquid or excessively frequent stools. [NIH]

Endothelium: The layer of epithelial cells that lines the cavities of the heart and of the blood and lymph vessels, and the serous cavities of the body, originating from the mesoderm. [EU]

Hormonal: Pertaining to or of the nature of a hormone. [EU]

Iodine: A nonmetallic element of the halogen group that is represented by the atomic symbol I, atomic number 53, and atomic weight of 126.90. It is a nutritionally essential element, especially important in thyroid hormone synthesis. In solution, it has anti-infective properties and is used topically. [NIH]

Lithium: Lithium. An element in the alkali metals family. It has the atomic symbol Li, atomic number 3, and atomic weight 6.94. Salts of lithium are used in treating manic-depressive disorders. [NIH]

Niacin: Water-soluble vitamin of the B complex occurring in various animal and plant tissues. Required by the body for the formation of coenzymes NAD and NADP. Has pellagra-curative, vasodilating, and antilipemic properties. [NIH]

Overdose: 1. to administer an excessive dose. 2. an excessive dose. [EU]

Riboflavin: Nutritional factor found in milk, eggs, malted barley, liver, kidney, heart, and leafy vegetables. The richest natural source is yeast. It occurs in the free form only in the retina of the eye, in whey, and in urine; its principal forms in tissues and cells are as FMN and FAD. [NIH]

Thyroxine: An amino acid of the thyroid gland which exerts a stimulating effect on thyroid metabolism. [NIH]

APPENDIX D. FINDING MEDICAL LIBRARIES

Overview

At a medical library you can find medical texts and reference books, consumer health publications, specialty newspapers and magazines, as well as medical journals. In this Appendix, we show you how to quickly find a medical library in your area.

Preparation

Before going to the library, highlight the references mentioned in this sourcebook that you find interesting. Focus on those items that are not available via the Internet, and ask the reference librarian for help with your search. He or she may know of additional resources that could be helpful to you. Most importantly, your local public library and medical libraries have Interlibrary Loan programs with the National Library of Medicine (NLM), one of the largest medical collections in the world. According to the NLM, most of the literature in the general and historical collections of the National Library of Medicine is available on interlibrary loan to any library. NLM's interlibrary loan services are only available to libraries. If you would like to access NLM medical literature, then visit a library in your area that can request the publications for you.[50]

---

[50] Adapted from the NLM: **http://www.nlm.nih.gov/psd/cas/interlibrary.html**

Finding a Local Medical Library

The quickest method to locate medical libraries is to use the Internet-based directory published by the National Network of Libraries of Medicine (NN/LM). This network includes 4626 members and affiliates that provide many services to librarians, health professionals, and the public. To find a library in your area, simply visit **http://nnlm.gov/members/adv.html** or call 1-800-338-7657.

Medical Libraries Open to the Public

In addition to the NN/LM, the National Library of Medicine (NLM) lists a number of libraries that are generally open to the public and have reference facilities. The following is the NLM's list plus hyperlinks to each library Web site. These Web pages can provide information on hours of operation and other restrictions. The list below is a small sample of libraries recommended by the National Library of Medicine (sorted alphabetically by name of the U.S. state or Canadian province where the library is located):[51]

- **Alabama:** Health InfoNet of Jefferson County (Jefferson County Library Cooperative, Lister Hill Library of the Health Sciences), **http://www.uab.edu/infonet/**

- **Alabama:** Richard M. Scrushy Library (American Sports Medicine Institute), **http://www.asmi.org/LIBRARY.HTM**

- **Arizona:** Samaritan Regional Medical Center: The Learning Center (Samaritan Health System, Phoenix, Arizona), **http://www.samaritan.edu/library/bannerlibs.htm**

- **California:** Kris Kelly Health Information Center (St. Joseph Health System), **http://www.humboldt1.com/~kkhic/index.html**

- **California:** Community Health Library of Los Gatos (Community Health Library of Los Gatos), **http://www.healthlib.org/orgresources.html**

- **California:** Consumer Health Program and Services (CHIPS) (County of Los Angeles Public Library, Los Angeles County Harbor-UCLA Medical Center Library) - Carson, CA, **http://www.colapublib.org/services/chips.html**

- **California:** Gateway Health Library (Sutter Gould Medical Foundation)

- **California:** Health Library (Stanford University Medical Center), **http://www-med.stanford.edu/healthlibrary/**

---

[51] Abstracted from **http://www.nlm.nih.gov/medlineplus/libraries.html**

- **California:** Patient Education Resource Center - Health Information and Resources (University of California, San Francisco), **http://sfghdean.ucsf.edu/barnett/PERC/default.asp**

- **California:** Redwood Health Library (Petaluma Health Care District), **http://www.phcd.org/rdwdlib.html**

- **California:** San José PlaneTree Health Library, **http://planetreesanjose.org/**

- **California:** Sutter Resource Library (Sutter Hospitals Foundation), **http://go.sutterhealth.org/comm/resc-library/sac-resources.html**

- **California:** University of California, Davis. Health Sciences Libraries

- **California:** ValleyCare Health Library & Ryan Comer Cancer Resource Center (ValleyCare Health System), **http://www.valleycare.com/library.html**

- **California:** Washington Community Health Resource Library (Washington Community Health Resource Library), **http://www.healthlibrary.org/**

- **Colorado:** William V. Gervasini Memorial Library (Exempla Healthcare), **http://www.exempla.org/conslib.htm**

- **Connecticut:** Hartford Hospital Health Science Libraries (Hartford Hospital), **http://www.harthosp.org/library/**

- **Connecticut:** Healthnet: Connecticut Consumer Health Information Center (University of Connecticut Health Center, Lyman Maynard Stowe Library), **http://library.uchc.edu/departm/hnet/**

- **Connecticut:** Waterbury Hospital Health Center Library (Waterbury Hospital), **http://www.waterburyhospital.com/library/consumer.shtml**

- **Delaware:** Consumer Health Library (Christiana Care Health System, Eugene du Pont Preventive Medicine & Rehabilitation Institute), **http://www.christianacare.org/health_guide/health_guide_pmri_health _info.cfm**

- **Delaware:** Lewis B. Flinn Library (Delaware Academy of Medicine), **http://www.delamed.org/chls.html**

- **Georgia:** Family Resource Library (Medical College of Georgia), **http://cmc.mcg.edu/kids_families/fam_resources/fam_res_lib/frl.htm**

- **Georgia:** Health Resource Center (Medical Center of Central Georgia), **http://www.mccg.org/hrc/hrchome.asp**

- **Hawaii:** Hawaii Medical Library: Consumer Health Information Service (Hawaii Medical Library), **http://hml.org/CHIS/**

- **Idaho:** DeArmond Consumer Health Library (Kootenai Medical Center), **http://www.nicon.org/DeArmond/index.htm**

- **Illinois:** Health Learning Center of Northwestern Memorial Hospital (Northwestern Memorial Hospital, Health Learning Center), **http://www.nmh.org/health_info/hlc.html**

- **Illinois:** Medical Library (OSF Saint Francis Medical Center), **http://www.osfsaintfrancis.org/general/library/**

- **Kentucky:** Medical Library - Services for Patients, Families, Students & the Public (Central Baptist Hospital), **http://www.centralbap.com/education/community/library.htm**

- **Kentucky:** University of Kentucky - Health Information Library (University of Kentucky, Chandler Medical Center, Health Information Library), **http://www.mc.uky.edu/PatientEd/**

- **Louisiana:** Alton Ochsner Medical Foundation Library (Alton Ochsner Medical Foundation), **http://www.ochsner.org/library/**

- **Louisiana:** Louisiana State University Health Sciences Center Medical Library-Shreveport, **http://lib-sh.lsuhsc.edu/**

- **Maine:** Franklin Memorial Hospital Medical Library (Franklin Memorial Hospital), **http://www.fchn.org/fmh/lib.htm**

- **Maine:** Gerrish-True Health Sciences Library (Central Maine Medical Center), **http://www.cmmc.org/library/library.html**

- **Maine:** Hadley Parrot Health Science Library (Eastern Maine Healthcare), **http://www.emh.org/hll/hpl/guide.htm**

- **Maine:** Maine Medical Center Library (Maine Medical Center), **http://www.mmc.org/library/**

- **Maine:** Parkview Hospital, **http://www.parkviewhospital.org/communit.htm#Library**

- **Maine:** Southern Maine Medical Center Health Sciences Library (Southern Maine Medical Center), **http://www.smmc.org/services/service.php3?choice=10**

- **Maine:** Stephens Memorial Hospital Health Information Library (Western Maine Health), **http://www.wmhcc.com/hil_frame.html**

- **Manitoba, Canada:** Consumer & Patient Health Information Service (University of Manitoba Libraries), **http://www.umanitoba.ca/libraries/units/health/reference/chis.html**

- **Manitoba, Canada:** J.W. Crane Memorial Library (Deer Lodge Centre), **http://www.deerlodge.mb.ca/library/libraryservices.shtml**

- **Maryland:** Health Information Center at the Wheaton Regional Library (Montgomery County, Md., Dept. of Public Libraries, Wheaton Regional Library), **http://www.mont.lib.md.us/healthinfo/hic.asp**

- **Massachusetts:** Baystate Medical Center Library (Baystate Health System), **http://www.baystatehealth.com/1024/**

- **Massachusetts:** Boston University Medical Center Alumni Medical Library (Boston University Medical Center), **http://med-libwww.bu.edu/library/lib.html**

- **Massachusetts:** Lowell General Hospital Health Sciences Library (Lowell General Hospital), **http://www.lowellgeneral.org/library/HomePageLinks/WWW.htm**

- **Massachusetts:** Paul E. Woodard Health Sciences Library (New England Baptist Hospital), **http://www.nebh.org/health_lib.asp**

- **Massachusetts:** St. Luke's Hospital Health Sciences Library (St. Luke's Hospital), **http://www.southcoast.org/library/**

- **Massachusetts:** Treadwell Library Consumer Health Reference Center (Massachusetts General Hospital), **http://www.mgh.harvard.edu/library/chrcindex.html**

- **Massachusetts:** UMass HealthNet (University of Massachusetts Medical School), **http://healthnet.umassmed.edu/**

- **Michigan:** Botsford General Hospital Library - Consumer Health (Botsford General Hospital, Library & Internet Services), **http://www.botsfordlibrary.org/consumer.htm**

- **Michigan:** Helen DeRoy Medical Library (Providence Hospital and Medical Centers), **http://www.providence-hospital.org/library/**

- **Michigan:** Marquette General Hospital - Consumer Health Library (Marquette General Hospital, Health Information Center), **http://www.mgh.org/center.html**

- **Michigan:** Patient Education Resouce Center - University of Michigan Cancer Center (University of Michigan Comprehensive Cancer Center), **http://www.cancer.med.umich.edu/learn/leares.htm**

- **Michigan:** Sladen Library & Center for Health Information Resources - Consumer Health Information, **http://www.sladen.hfhs.org/library/consumer/index.html**

- **Montana:** Center for Health Information (St. Patrick Hospital and Health Sciences Center), **http://www.saintpatrick.org/chi/librarydetail.php3?ID=41**

- **National:** Consumer Health Library Directory (Medical Library Association, Consumer and Patient Health Information Section), **http://caphis.mlanet.org/directory/index.html**

- **National:** National Network of Libraries of Medicine (National Library of Medicine) - provides library services for health professionals in the United States who do not have access to a medical library, **http://nnlm.gov/**

- **National:** NN/LM List of Libraries Serving the Public (National Network of Libraries of Medicine), **http://nnlm.gov/members/**

- **Nevada:** Health Science Library, West Charleston Library (Las Vegas Clark County Library District), **http://www.lvccld.org/special_collections/medical/index.htm**

- **New Hampshire:** Dartmouth Biomedical Libraries (Dartmouth College Library), **http://www.dartmouth.edu/~biomed/resources.htmld/conshealth.htmld/**

- **New Jersey:** Consumer Health Library (Rahway Hospital), **http://www.rahwayhospital.com/library.htm**

- **New Jersey:** Dr. Walter Phillips Health Sciences Library (Englewood Hospital and Medical Center), **http://www.englewoodhospital.com/links/index.htm**

- **New Jersey:** Meland Foundation (Englewood Hospital and Medical Center), **http://www.geocities.com/ResearchTriangle/9360/**

- **New York:** Choices in Health Information (New York Public Library) - NLM Consumer Pilot Project participant, **http://www.nypl.org/branch/health/links.html**

- **New York:** Health Information Center (Upstate Medical University, State University of New York), **http://www.upstate.edu/library/hic/**

- **New York:** Health Sciences Library (Long Island Jewish Medical Center), **http://www.lij.edu/library/library.html**

- **New York:** ViaHealth Medical Library (Rochester General Hospital), **http://www.nyam.org/library/**

- **Ohio:** Consumer Health Library (Akron General Medical Center, Medical & Consumer Health Library), **http://www.akrongeneral.org/hwlibrary.htm**

- **Oklahoma:** Saint Francis Health System Patient/Family Resource Center (Saint Francis Health System), **http://www.sfh-tulsa.com/patientfamilycenter/default.asp**

- **Oregon:** Planetree Health Resource Center (Mid-Columbia Medical Center), **http://www.mcmc.net/phrc/**

- **Pennsylvania:** Community Health Information Library (Milton S. Hershey Medical Center), **http://www.hmc.psu.edu/commhealth/**

- **Pennsylvania:** Community Health Resource Library (Geisinger Medical Center), **http://www.geisinger.edu/education/commlib.shtml**

- **Pennsylvania:** HealthInfo Library (Moses Taylor Hospital), **http://www.mth.org/healthwellness.html**

- **Pennsylvania:** Hopwood Library (University of Pittsburgh, Health Sciences Library System), **http://www.hsls.pitt.edu/chi/hhrcinfo.html**

- **Pennsylvania:** Koop Community Health Information Center (College of Physicians of Philadelphia), **http://www.collphyphil.org/kooppg1.shtml**

- **Pennsylvania:** Learning Resources Center - Medical Library (Susquehanna Health System), **http://www.shscares.org/services/lrc/index.asp**

- **Pennsylvania:** Medical Library (UPMC Health System), **http://www.upmc.edu/passavant/library.htm**

- **Quebec, Canada:** Medical Library (Montreal General Hospital), **http://ww2.mcgill.ca/mghlib/**

- **South Dakota:** Rapid City Regional Hospital - Health Information Center (Rapid City Regional Hospital, Health Information Center), **http://www.rcrh.org/education/LibraryResourcesConsumers.htm**

- **Texas:** Houston HealthWays (Houston Academy of Medicine-Texas Medical Center Library), **http://hhw.library.tmc.edu/**

- **Texas:** Matustik Family Resource Center (Cook Children's Health Care System), **http://www.cookchildrens.com/Matustik_Library.html**

- **Washington:** Community Health Library (Kittitas Valley Community Hospital), **http://www.kvch.com/**

- **Washington:** Southwest Washington Medical Center Library (Southwest Washington Medical Center), **http://www.swmedctr.com/Home/**

APPENDIX E. YOUR RIGHTS AND INSURANCE

Overview

Any patient with polycystic kidney disease faces a series of issues related more to the healthcare industry than to the medical condition itself. This appendix covers two important topics in this regard: your rights and responsibilities as a patient, and how to get the most out of your medical insurance plan.

Your Rights as a Patient

The President's Advisory Commission on Consumer Protection and Quality in the Healthcare Industry has created the following summary of your rights as a patient.[52]

Information Disclosure

Consumers have the right to receive accurate, easily understood information. Some consumers require assistance in making informed decisions about health plans, health professionals, and healthcare facilities. Such information includes:

- *Health plans.* Covered benefits, cost-sharing, and procedures for resolving complaints, licensure, certification, and accreditation status, comparable measures of quality and consumer satisfaction, provider

---

[52]Adapted from Consumer Bill of Rights and Responsibilities: **http://www.hcqualitycommission.gov/press/cbor.html#head1**.

network composition, the procedures that govern access to specialists and emergency services, and care management information.

- *Health professionals.* Education, board certification, and recertification, years of practice, experience performing certain procedures, and comparable measures of quality and consumer satisfaction.

- *Healthcare facilities.* Experience in performing certain procedures and services, accreditation status, comparable measures of quality, worker, and consumer satisfaction, and procedures for resolving complaints.

- *Consumer assistance programs.* Programs must be carefully structured to promote consumer confidence and to work cooperatively with health plans, providers, payers, and regulators. Desirable characteristics of such programs are sponsorship that ensures accountability to the interests of consumers and stable, adequate funding.

Choice of Providers and Plans

Consumers have the right to a choice of healthcare providers that is sufficient to ensure access to appropriate high-quality healthcare. To ensure such choice, the Commission recommends the following:

- *Provider network adequacy.* All health plan networks should provide access to sufficient numbers and types of providers to assure that all covered services will be accessible without unreasonable delay -- including access to emergency services 24 hours a day and 7 days a week. If a health plan has an insufficient number or type of providers to provide a covered benefit with the appropriate degree of specialization, the plan should ensure that the consumer obtains the benefit outside the network at no greater cost than if the benefit were obtained from participating providers.

- *Women's health services.* Women should be able to choose a qualified provider offered by a plan -- such as gynecologists, certified nurse midwives, and other qualified healthcare providers -- for the provision of covered care necessary to provide routine and preventative women's healthcare services.

- *Access to specialists.* Consumers with complex or serious medical conditions who require frequent specialty care should have direct access to a qualified specialist of their choice within a plan's network of providers. Authorizations, when required, should be for an adequate number of direct access visits under an approved treatment plan.

- *Transitional care.* Consumers who are undergoing a course of treatment for a chronic or disabling condition (or who are in the second or third trimester of a pregnancy) at the time they involuntarily change health plans or at a time when a provider is terminated by a plan for other than cause should be able to continue seeing their current specialty providers for up to 90 days (or through completion of postpartum care) to allow for transition of care.

- *Choice of health plans.* Public and private group purchasers should, wherever feasible, offer consumers a choice of high-quality health insurance plans.

Access to Emergency Services

Consumers have the right to access emergency healthcare services when and where the need arises. Health plans should provide payment when a consumer presents to an emergency department with acute symptoms of sufficient severity--including severe pain--such that a "prudent layperson" could reasonably expect the absence of medical attention to result in placing that consumer's health in serious jeopardy, serious impairment to bodily functions, or serious dysfunction of any bodily organ or part.

Participation in Treatment Decisions

Consumers have the right and responsibility to fully participate in all decisions related to their healthcare. Consumers who are unable to fully participate in treatment decisions have the right to be represented by parents, guardians, family members, or other conservators. Physicians and other health professionals should:

- Provide patients with sufficient information and opportunity to decide among treatment options consistent with the informed consent process.

- Discuss all treatment options with a patient in a culturally competent manner, including the option of no treatment at all.

- Ensure that persons with disabilities have effective communications with members of the health system in making such decisions.

- Discuss all current treatments a consumer may be undergoing.

- Discuss all risks, benefits, and consequences to treatment or nontreatment.

- Give patients the opportunity to refuse treatment and to express preferences about future treatment decisions.

- Discuss the use of advance directives -- both living wills and durable powers of attorney for healthcare -- with patients and their designated family members.

- Abide by the decisions made by their patients and/or their designated representatives consistent with the informed consent process.

Health plans, health providers, and healthcare facilities should:

- Disclose to consumers factors -- such as methods of compensation, ownership of or interest in healthcare facilities, or matters of conscience -- that could influence advice or treatment decisions.

- Assure that provider contracts do not contain any so-called "gag clauses" or other contractual mechanisms that restrict healthcare providers' ability to communicate with and advise patients about medically necessary treatment options.

- Be prohibited from penalizing or seeking retribution against healthcare professionals or other health workers for advocating on behalf of their patients.

Respect and Nondiscrimination

Consumers have the right to considerate, respectful care from all members of the healthcare industry at all times and under all circumstances. An environment of mutual respect is essential to maintain a quality healthcare system. To assure that right, the Commission recommends the following:

- Consumers must not be discriminated against in the delivery of healthcare services consistent with the benefits covered in their policy, or as required by law, based on race, ethnicity, national origin, religion, sex, age, mental or physical disability, sexual orientation, genetic information, or source of payment.

- Consumers eligible for coverage under the terms and conditions of a health plan or program, or as required by law, must not be discriminated against in marketing and enrollment practices based on race, ethnicity, national origin, religion, sex, age, mental or physical disability, sexual orientation, genetic information, or source of payment.

Confidentiality of Health Information

Consumers have the right to communicate with healthcare providers in confidence and to have the confidentiality of their individually identifiable healthcare information protected. Consumers also have the right to review and copy their own medical records and request amendments to their records.

Complaints and Appeals

Consumers have the right to a fair and efficient process for resolving differences with their health plans, healthcare providers, and the institutions that serve them, including a rigorous system of internal review and an independent system of external review. A free copy of the Patient's Bill of Rights is available from the American Hospital Association.[53]

Patient Responsibilities

Treatment is a two-way street between you and your healthcare providers. To underscore the importance of finance in modern healthcare as well as your responsibility for the financial aspects of your care, the President's Advisory Commission on Consumer Protection and Quality in the Healthcare Industry has proposed that patients understand the following "Consumer Responsibilities."[54] In a healthcare system that protects consumers' rights, it is reasonable to expect and encourage consumers to assume certain responsibilities. Greater individual involvement by the consumer in his or her care increases the likelihood of achieving the best outcome and helps support a quality-oriented, cost-conscious environment. Such responsibilities include:

- Take responsibility for maximizing healthy habits such as exercising, not smoking, and eating a healthy diet.

- Work collaboratively with healthcare providers in developing and carrying out agreed-upon treatment plans.

- Disclose relevant information and clearly communicate wants and needs.

---

[53] To order your free copy of the Patient's Bill of Rights, telephone 312-422-3000 or visit the American Hospital Association's Web site: **http://www.aha.org**. Click on "Resource Center," go to "Search" at bottom of page, and then type in "Patient's Bill of Rights." The Patient's Bill of Rights is also available from Fax on Demand, at 312-422-2020, document number 471124.

[54] Adapted from **http://www.hcqualitycommission.gov/press/cbor.html#head1**.

- Use your health insurance plan's internal complaint and appeal processes to address your concerns.

- Avoid knowingly spreading disease.

- Recognize the reality of risks, the limits of the medical science, and the human fallibility of the healthcare professional.

- Be aware of a healthcare provider's obligation to be reasonably efficient and equitable in providing care to other patients and the community.

- Become knowledgeable about your health plan's coverage and options (when available) including all covered benefits, limitations, and exclusions, rules regarding use of network providers, coverage and referral rules, appropriate processes to secure additional information, and the process to appeal coverage decisions.

- Show respect for other patients and health workers.

- Make a good-faith effort to meet financial obligations.

- Abide by administrative and operational procedures of health plans, healthcare providers, and Government health benefit programs.

Choosing an Insurance Plan

There are a number of official government agencies that help consumers understand their healthcare insurance choices.[55] The U.S. Department of Labor, in particular, recommends ten ways to make your health benefits choices work best for you.[56]

1. Your options are important. There are many different types of health benefit plans. Find out which one your employer offers, then check out the plan, or plans, offered. Your employer's human resource office, the health plan administrator, or your union can provide information to help you match your needs and preferences with the available plans. The more information you have, the better your healthcare decisions will be.

2. Reviewing the benefits available. Do the plans offered cover preventive care, well-baby care, vision or dental care? Are there deductibles? Answers to these questions can help determine the out-of-pocket expenses you may

---

[55] More information about quality across programs is provided at the following AHRQ Web site:
http://www.ahrq.gov/consumer/qntascii/qnthplan.htm .
[56] Adapted from the Department of Labor:
http://www.dol.gov/dol/pwba/public/pubs/health/top10-text.html.

face. Matching your needs and those of your family members will result in the best possible benefits. Cheapest may not always be best. Your goal is high quality health benefits.

3. Look for quality. The quality of healthcare services varies, but quality can be measured. You should consider the quality of healthcare in deciding among the healthcare plans or options available to you. Not all health plans, doctors, hospitals and other providers give the highest quality care. Fortunately, there is quality information you can use right now to help you compare your healthcare choices. Find out how you can measure quality. Consult the U.S. Department of Health and Human Services publication "Your Guide to Choosing Quality Health Care" on the Internet at **www.ahcpr.gov/consumer**.

4. Your plan's summary plan description (SPD) provides a wealth of information. Your health plan administrator can provide you with a copy of your plan's SPD. It outlines your benefits and your legal rights under the Employee Retirement Income Security Act (ERISA), the federal law that protects your health benefits. It should contain information about the coverage of dependents, what services will require a co-pay, and the circumstances under which your employer can change or terminate a health benefits plan. Save the SPD and all other health plan brochures and documents, along with memos or correspondence from your employer relating to health benefits.

5. Assess your benefit coverage as your family status changes. Marriage, divorce, childbirth or adoption, and the death of a spouse are all life events that may signal a need to change your health benefits. You, your spouse and dependent children may be eligible for a special enrollment period under provisions of the Health Insurance Portability and Accountability Act (HIPAA). Even without life-changing events, the information provided by your employer should tell you how you can change benefits or switch plans, if more than one plan is offered. If your spouse's employer also offers a health benefits package, consider coordinating both plans for maximum coverage.

6. Changing jobs and other life events can affect your health benefits. Under the Consolidated Omnibus Budget Reconciliation Act (COBRA), you, your covered spouse, and your dependent children may be eligible to purchase extended health coverage under your employer's plan if you lose your job, change employers, get divorced, or upon occurrence of certain other events. Coverage can range from 18 to 36 months depending on your situation. COBRA applies to most employers with 20 or more workers and requires your plan to notify you of your rights. Most plans require eligible individuals to make their COBRA election within 60 days of the plan's notice. Be sure to follow up with your plan sponsor if you don't receive notice, and make sure you respond within the allotted time.

7. HIPAA can also help if you are changing jobs, particularly if you have a medical condition. HIPAA generally limits pre-existing condition exclusions to a maximum of 12 months (18 months for late enrollees). HIPAA also requires this maximum period to be reduced by the length of time you had prior "creditable coverage." You should receive a certificate documenting your prior creditable coverage from your old plan when coverage ends.

8. Plan for retirement. Before you retire, find out what health benefits, if any, extend to you and your spouse during your retirement years. Consult with your employer's human resources office, your union, the plan administrator, and check your SPD. Make sure there is no conflicting information among these sources about the benefits you will receive or the circumstances under which they can change or be eliminated. With this information in hand, you can make other important choices, like finding out if you are eligible for Medicare and Medigap insurance coverage.

9. Know how to file an appeal if your health benefits daim is denied. Understand how your plan handles grievances and where to make appeals of the plan's decisions. Keep records and copies of correspondence. Check your health benefits package and your SPD to determine who is responsible for handling problems with benefit claims. Contact PWBA for customer service assistance if you are unable to obtain a response to your complaint.

10. You can take steps to improve the quality of the healthcare and the health benefits you receive. Look for and use things like Quality Reports and Accreditation Reports whenever you can. Quality reports may contain consumer ratings -- how satisfied consumers are with the doctors in their plan, for instance-- and clinical performance measures -- how well a healthcare organization prevents and treats illness. Accreditation reports provide information on how accredited organizations meet national standards, and often include clinical performance measures. Look for these quality measures whenever possible. Consult "Your Guide to Choosing Quality Health Care" on the Internet at **www.ahcpr.gov/consumer**.

Medicare and Medicaid

Illness strikes both rich and poor families. For low-income families, Medicaid is available to defer the costs of treatment. The Health Care Financing Administration (HCFA) administers Medicare, the nation's largest health insurance program, which covers 39 million Americans. In the following pages, you will learn the basics about Medicare insurance as well as useful contact information on how to find more in-depth information about Medicaid.[57]

Who is Eligible for Medicare?

Generally, you are eligible for Medicare if you or your spouse worked for at least 10 years in Medicare-covered employment and you are 65 years old and a citizen or permanent resident of the United States. You might also qualify for coverage if you are under age 65 but have a disability or End-Stage Renal disease (permanent kidney failure requiring dialysis or transplant). Here are some simple guidelines:

You can get Part A at age 65 without having to pay premiums if:

- You are already receiving retirement benefits from Social Security or the Railroad Retirement Board.

- You are eligible to receive Social Security or Railroad benefits but have not yet filed for them.

- You or your spouse had Medicare-covered government employment.

If you are under 65, you can get Part A without having to pay premiums if:

- You have received Social Security or Railroad Retirement Board disability benefit for 24 months.

- You are a kidney dialysis or kidney transplant patient.

Medicare has two parts:

- Part A (Hospital Insurance). Most people do not have to pay for Part A.
- Part B (Medical Insurance). Most people pay monthly for Part B.

---

[57] This section has been adapted from the Official U.S. Site for Medicare Information: **http://www.medicare.gov/Basics/Overview.asp**.

Part A (Hospital Insurance)

Helps Pay For: Inpatient hospital care, care in critical access hospitals (small facilities that give limited outpatient and inpatient services to people in rural areas) and skilled nursing facilities, hospice care, and some home healthcare.

Cost: Most people get Part A automatically when they turn age 65. You do not have to pay a monthly payment called a premium for Part A because you or a spouse paid Medicare taxes while you were working.

If you (or your spouse) did not pay Medicare taxes while you were working and you are age 65 or older, you still may be able to buy Part A. If you are not sure you have Part A, look on your red, white, and blue Medicare card. It will show "Hospital Part A" on the lower left corner of the card. You can also call the Social Security Administration toll free at 1-800-772-1213 or call your local Social Security office for more information about buying Part A. If you get benefits from the Railroad Retirement Board, call your local RRB office or 1-800-808-0772. For more information, call your Fiscal Intermediary about Part A bills and services. The phone number for the Fiscal Intermediary office in your area can be obtained from the following Web site: **http://www.medicare.gov/Contacts/home.asp**.

Part B (Medical Insurance)

Helps Pay For: Doctors, services, outpatient hospital care, and some other medical services that Part A does not cover, such as the services of physical and occupational therapists, and some home healthcare. Part B helps pay for covered services and supplies when they are medically necessary.

Cost: As of 2001, you pay the Medicare Part B premium of $50.00 per month. In some cases this amount may be higher if you did not choose Part B when you first became eligible at age 65. The cost of Part B may go up 10% for each 12-month period that you were eligible for Part B but declined coverage, except in special cases. You will have to pay the extra 10% cost for the rest of your life.

Enrolling in Part B is your choice. You can sign up for Part B anytime during a 7-month period that begins 3 months before you turn 65. Visit your local Social Security office, or call the Social Security Administration at 1-800-772-1213 to sign up. If you choose to enroll in Part B, the premium is usually taken out of your monthly Social Security, Railroad Retirement, or Civil Service Retirement payment. If you do not receive any of the above payments, Medicare sends you a bill for your part B premium every 3 months. You should receive your Medicare premium bill in the mail by the 10th of the month. If you do not, call the Social Security Administration at 1-800-772-1213, or your local Social Security office. If you get benefits from the Railroad Retirement Board, call your local RRB office or 1-800-808-0772. For more information, call your Medicare carrier about bills and services. The phone number for the Medicare carrier in your area can be found at the following Web site: **http://www.medicare.gov/Contacts/home.asp**. You may have choices in how you get your healthcare including the Original Medicare Plan, Medicare Managed Care Plans (like HMOs), and Medicare Private Fee-for-Service Plans.

Medicaid

Medicaid is a joint federal and state program that helps pay medical costs for some people with low incomes and limited resources. Medicaid programs vary from state to state. People on Medicaid may also get coverage for nursing home care and outpatient prescription drugs which are not covered by Medicare. You can find more information about Medicaid on the HCFA.gov Web site at **http://www.hcfa.gov/medicaid/medicaid.htm**.

States also have programs that pay some or all of Medicare's premiums and may also pay Medicare deductibles and coinsurance for certain people who have Medicare and a low income. To qualify, you must have:

- Part A (Hospital Insurance),

- Assets, such as bank accounts, stocks, and bonds that are not more than $4,000 for a single person, or $6,000 for a couple, and

- A monthly income that is below certain limits.

For more information on these programs, look at the Medicare Savings Programs brochure, **http://www.medicare.gov/Library/PDFNavigation/PDFInterim.asp?Language=English&Type=Pub&PubID=10126**. There are also Prescription Drug Assistance Programs available. Find information on these programs which offer discounts or free medications to individuals in need at **http://www.medicare.gov/Prescription/Home.asp**.

NORD's Medication Assistance Programs

Finally, the National Organization for Rare Disorders, Inc. (NORD) administers medication programs sponsored by humanitarian-minded pharmaceutical and biotechnology companies to help uninsured or under-insured individuals secure life-saving or life-sustaining drugs.[58] NORD programs ensure that certain vital drugs are available "to those individuals whose income is too high to qualify for Medicaid but too low to pay for their prescribed medications." The program has standards for fairness, equity, and unbiased eligibility. It currently covers some 14 programs for nine pharmaceutical companies. NORD also offers early access programs for investigational new drugs (IND) under the approved "Treatment INDs" programs of the Food and Drug Administration (FDA). In these programs, a limited number of individuals can receive investigational drugs that have yet to be approved by the FDA. These programs are generally designed for rare diseases or disorders. For more information, visit **www.rarediseases.org**.

Additional Resources

In addition to the references already listed in this chapter, you may need more information on health insurance, hospitals, or the healthcare system in general. The NIH has set up an excellent guidance Web site that addresses these and other issues. Topics include:[59]

- Health Insurance:
  http://www.nlm.nih.gov/medlineplus/healthinsurance.html

- Health Statistics:
  http://www.nlm.nih.gov/medlineplus/healthstatistics.html

- HMO and Managed Care:
  http://www.nlm.nih.gov/medlineplus/managedcare.html

- Hospice Care: **http://www.nlm.nih.gov/medlineplus/hospicecare.html**

- Medicaid: **http://www.nlm.nih.gov/medlineplus/medicaid.html**

- Medicare: **http://www.nlm.nih.gov/medlineplus/medicare.html**

- Nursing Homes and Long-term Care:
  http://www.nlm.nih.gov/medlineplus/nursinghomes.html

---

[58] Adapted from NORD: **http://www.rarediseases.org/cgi-bin/nord/progserv#patient?id=rPIzL9oD&mv_pc=30**.

[59] You can access this information at:
http://www.nlm.nih.gov/medlineplus/healthsystem.html.

- Patient's Rights, Confidentiality, Informed Consent, Ombudsman Programs, Privacy and Patient Issues: **http://www.nlm.nih.gov/medlineplus/patientissues.html**

- Veteran's Health, Persian Gulf War, Gulf War Syndrome, Agent Orange: **http://www.nlm.nih.gov/medlineplus/veteranshealth.html**

APPENDIX F. ANEMIA IN KIDNEY DISEASE

Overview[60]

If your blood is low in red blood cells, you have anemia. Red blood cells carry oxygen (O_2) to tissues and organs throughout your body and enable them to use the energy from food. Without oxygen, these tissues and organs--particularly the heart and brain--may not do their jobs as well as they should. For this reason, if you have anemia, you may tire easily and look pale. Anemia may also contribute to heart problems.

Anemia is common in people with kidney disease. Healthy kidneys produce a hormone called erythropoietin, or EPO, which stimulates the bone marrow to produce the proper number of red blood cells needed to carry oxygen to vital organs. Diseased kidneys, however, often don't make enough EPO. As a result, the bone marrow makes fewer red blood cells. Other common causes of anemia include loss of blood from hemodialysis and low levels of iron and folic acid. These nutrients from food help young red blood cells make hemoglobin (Hgb), their main oxygen-carrying protein.

---

[60] Adapted from the National Institute of Diabetes and Digestive and Kidney Diseases (NIDDK): **http://www.niddk.nih.gov/health/kidney/pubs/kidney-failure/anemia/anemia.htm**.

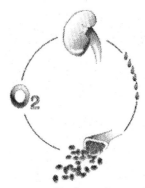

Healthy kidneys produce a hormone called erythropoietin, or EPO, which stimulates the bone marrow to make red blood cells needed to carry oxygen (O₂) throughout the body.

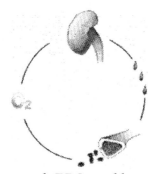

Diseased kidneys don't make enough EPO, and bone marrow then makes fewer red blood cells.

Laboratory Tests

A complete blood count (CBC), a laboratory test performed on a sample of your blood, includes a determination of your hematocrit (Hct), the percentage of the blood that consists of red blood cells. The CBC also measures the amount of Hgb in your blood. The range of normal Hct and Hgb in women who menstruate is slightly lower than for healthy men or healthy postmenopausal women. The Hgb is usually about one-third the value of the Hct.

When Anemia Begins

Anemia may begin to develop in the early stages of kidney disease, when you still have 20 percent to 50 percent of your normal kidney function. This partial loss of kidney function is often called chronic renal insufficiency.

Anemia tends to worsen as kidney disease progresses. End-stage kidney failure, the point at which dialysis or kidney transplantation becomes necessary, doesn't occur until you have only about 10 percent of your kidney function remaining. Nearly everyone with end-stage kidney failure has anemia.

Diagnosis

If you have lost at least half of normal kidney function (serum creatinine greater than 2 mg/dL) and have a low Hct, the most likely cause of anemia is decreased EPO production. The National Kidney Foundation's Dialysis Outcomes Quality Initiative (DOQI) recommends that doctors begin a detailed evaluation of anemia in men and postmenopausal women on dialysis when the Hct value falls below 37 percent. For women of childbearing age, evaluation should begin when the Hct falls below 33 percent. The evaluation will include tests for iron deficiency and blood loss in the stool to be certain there are no other reasons for the anemia.

When to Evaluate Dialysis Patients for Anemia[61]

	Hematocrit (Hct)	Hemoglobin (Hgb)
Women who menstruate	less than 33%	less than 11 g/dL
Men & postmenopausal women	less than 37%	less than 12 g/dL

Treatment

EPO

If no other cause for EPO deficiency is found, it can be treated with a genetically engineered form of the hormone, which is usually injected under the skin two or three times a week. Hemodialysis patients who can't tolerate EPO shots may receive the hormone intravenously during treatment, but this method requires a larger, more expensive dose and may not be as effective. DOQI recommends that patients treated with EPO therapy should achieve a target Hgb of 11 to 12 g/dL.

---

[61] Source: The National Kidney Foundation's Dialysis Outcomes Quality Initiative.

Iron

Many people with kidney disease need both EPO and iron supplements to raise their Hct to a satisfactory level. If your iron levels are too low, then EPO won't help and you'll continue to experience the effects of anemia. You may be able to take an iron pill, but many studies show that iron pills don't work as well in people with kidney failure as iron given intravenously. Iron is injected directly into an arm or into the tube that returns blood to your body during hemodialysis.

A nurse or doctor will give you a test dose because a very small number of people (less than 1 percent) have a bad reaction to iron injections. If you begin to wheeze or have trouble breathing, your health care provider can administer epinephrine or corticosteroids to counter the reaction. Even though the risk is small, you'll be asked to sign a form stating that you understand the possible reaction and that you agree to have the treatment. Talk with your health care provider if you have any questions.

In addition to measuring your Hct and Hgb, your tests will also include two measurements to show whether you have enough iron.

- Your ferritin level indicates the amount of iron stored in your body. According to DOQI guidelines, your ferritin score should be no less than 100 micrograms per liter (mcg/L) and no more than 800 mcg/L.

- TSAT stands for transferrin saturation, a score that indicates how much iron is available to make red blood cells. DOQI guidelines call for a TSAT score between 20 percent and 50 percent.

Other Causes of Anemia

In addition to EPO and iron, a few people may also need vitamin B_{12} and folic acid supplements.

If EPO, iron, vitamin B_{12}, and folic acid all fail, your doctor should look for other causes such as sickle cell disease or an inflammatory problem. At one time, aluminum poisoning contributed to anemia in people with kidney failure because many phosphate binders used for treating bone disease caused by kidney failure were antacids that contained aluminum. But aluminum-free alternatives are now widely available. Be sure your phosphate binder and your other drugs are free of aluminum.

Anemia keeps many people with kidney disease from feeling their best. But EPO treatments help most patients raise their Hgb, feel better, live longer, and have more energy.

Hope through Research

The National Institute of Diabetes and Digestive and Kidney Diseases (NIDDK), through its Division of Kidney, Urologic, and Hematologic Diseases, supports several programs and studies devoted to improving treatment for patients with progressive kidney disease and end-stage kidney failure (sometimes called end-stage renal disease, or ESRD), including patients on hemodialysis:

The End-Stage Renal Disease Program

This program promotes research to reduce medical problems from bone, blood, nervous system, metabolic, gastrointestinal, cardiovascular, and endocrine abnormalities in end-stage kidney failure and to improve the effectiveness of dialysis and transplantation. The research focuses on reuse of hemodialysis membranes and on using alternative dialyzer sterilization methods; on devising more efficient, biocompatible membranes; on refining high-flux hemodialysis; and on developing criteria for dialysis adequacy. The program also seeks to increase kidney graft and patient survival and to maximize quality of life.

The HEMO Study

This multicenter clinical trial is testing whether a higher hemodialysis dose and/or high-flux membranes will reduce patient mortality (death) and morbidity (medical problems).

The U.S. Renal Data System (USRDS)

This national data system collects, analyzes, and distributes information about the use of dialysis and transplantation to treat kidney failure in the United States. The USRDS is funded directly by the NIDDK in conjunction with the Health Care Financing Administration. The USRDS publishes an Annual Data Report, which characterizes the total population of people being treated for kidney failure; reports on incidence, prevalence, mortality rates, and trends over time; and develops data on the effects of various treatment modalities. The report also helps identify problems and opportunities for more focused special studies of renal research issues.

The Hemodialysis Vascular Access Clinical Trials Consortium

The Hemodialysis Vascular Access Clinical Trials Consortium will conduct a series of multicenter, randomized, placebo-controlled clinical trials of drug therapies to reduce the failure and complication rate of arteriovenous grafts and fistulas in hemodialysis. Recently developed antithrombotic agents and drugs to inhibit cytokines may be evaluated in these large clinical trials.

For More Information

For more information, contact the following organizations:

American Association of Kidney Patients
100 South Ashley Drive
Suite 280
Tampa, FL 33602
Phone: 1-800-749-2257 or (813) 223-7099
Fax: (813) 223-0001
Email: AAKPnat@aol.com
Internet: **www.aakp.org**

American Kidney Fund
6110 Executive Boulevard
Suite 1010
Rockville, MD 20852
Phone: 1-800-638-8299
Fax: (301) 881-0898
Email: helpline@akfinc.org
Internet: **www.akfinc.org**

National Kidney Foundation
30 East 33rd Street
New York, NY 10016
Phone: 1-800-622-9010
Fax: (212) 889-2210
Email: info@kidney.org

Internet: **www.kidney.org**

National Kidney and Urologic Diseases Information Clearinghouse
3 Information Way
Bethesda, MD 20892-3580
Email: nkudic@info.niddk.nih.gov
The National Kidney and Urologic Diseases Information Clearinghouse (NKUDIC) is a service of the National Institute of Diabetes and Digestive and Kidney Diseases (NIDDK). The NIDDK is part of the National Institutes of Health under the U.S. Department of Health and Human Services. Established in 1987, the clearinghouse provides information about diseases of the kidneys and urologic system to people with kidney and urologic disorders and to their families, health care professionals, and the public. NKUDIC answers inquiries, develops and distributes publications, and works closely with professional and patient organizations and Government agencies to coordinate resources about kidney and urologic diseases. Publications produced by the clearinghouse are carefully reviewed by both NIDDK scientists and outside experts. This fact sheet was reviewed by Dr. John C. Stivelman, Emory University School of Medicine.

ONLINE GLOSSARIES

The Internet provides access to a number of free-to-use medical dictionaries and glossaries. The National Library of Medicine has compiled the following list of online dictionaries:

- ADAM Medical Encyclopedia (A.D.A.M., Inc.), comprehensive medical reference: **http://www.nlm.nih.gov/medlineplus/encyclopedia.html**

- MedicineNet.com Medical Dictionary (MedicineNet, Inc.): **http://www.medterms.com/Script/Main/hp.asp**

- Merriam-Webster Medical Dictionary (Inteli-Health, Inc.): **http://www.intelihealth.com/IH/**

- Multilingual Glossary of Technical and Popular Medical Terms in Eight European Languages (European Commission) - Danish, Dutch, English, French, German, Italian, Portuguese, and Spanish: **http://allserv.rug.ac.be/~rvdstich/eugloss/welcome.html**

- On-line Medical Dictionary (CancerWEB): **http://www.graylab.ac.uk/omd/**

- Technology Glossary (National Library of Medicine) - Health Care Technology: **http://www.nlm.nih.gov/nichsr/ta101/ta10108.htm**

- Terms and Definitions (Office of Rare Diseases): **http://rarediseases.info.nih.gov/ord/glossary_a-e.html**

Beyond these, MEDLINEplus contains a very user-friendly encyclopedia covering every aspect of medicine (licensed from A.D.A.M., Inc.). The ADAM Medical Encyclopedia Web site address is **http://www.nlm.nih.gov/medlineplus/encyclopedia.html**. ADAM is also available on commercial Web sites such as Web MD (**http://my.webmd.com/adam/asset/adam_disease_articles/a_to_z/a**) and drkoop.com (**http://www.drkoop.com/**). Topics of interest can be researched by using keywords before continuing elsewhere, as these basic definitions and concepts will be useful in more advanced areas of research. You may choose to print various pages specifically relating to polycystic kidney disease and keep them on file. The NIH, in particular, suggests that patients with polycystic kidney disease visit the following Web sites in the ADAM Medical Encyclopedia:

- **Basic Guidelines for Polycystic Kidney Disease**

Hypertension
Web site:
http://www.nlm.nih.gov/medlineplus/ency/article/000468.htm

Kidney stones
Web site:
http://www.nlm.nih.gov/medlineplus/ency/article/000458.htm

PCKD
Web site:
http://www.nlm.nih.gov/medlineplus/ency/article/000502.htm

Polycystic kidney disease
Web site:
http://www.nlm.nih.gov/medlineplus/ency/article/000502.htm

- **Signs & Symptoms for Polycystic Kidney Disease**

Abdominal mass
Web site:
http://www.nlm.nih.gov/medlineplus/ency/article/003274.htm

Abdominal pain
Web site:
http://www.nlm.nih.gov/medlineplus/ency/article/003120.htm

Abdominal tenderness
Web site:
http://www.nlm.nih.gov/medlineplus/ency/article/003120.htm

Anemia
Web site:
http://www.nlm.nih.gov/medlineplus/ency/article/000560.htm

Blood in the urine
Web site:
http://www.nlm.nih.gov/medlineplus/ency/article/003138.htm

Cysts
Web site:
http://www.nlm.nih.gov/medlineplus/ency/article/003240.htm

Drowsiness
Web site:
http://www.nlm.nih.gov/medlineplus/ency/article/003208.htm

Dysuria
Web site:
http://www.nlm.nih.gov/medlineplus/ency/article/003145.htm

Enlarged liver
Web site:
http://www.nlm.nih.gov/medlineplus/ency/article/003275.htm

Excessive urination at night
Web site:
http://www.nlm.nih.gov/medlineplus/ency/article/003141.htm

Flank pain
Web site:
http://www.nlm.nih.gov/medlineplus/ency/article/003113.htm

Headache
Web site:
http://www.nlm.nih.gov/medlineplus/ency/article/003024.htm

Heart murmurs
Web site:
http://www.nlm.nih.gov/medlineplus/ency/article/003266.htm

Hematuria
Web site:
http://www.nlm.nih.gov/medlineplus/ency/article/003138.htm

Hepatomegaly
Web site:
http://www.nlm.nih.gov/medlineplus/ency/article/003275.htm

High blood pressure
Web site:
http://www.nlm.nih.gov/medlineplus/ency/article/003082.htm

Joint pain
Web site:
http://www.nlm.nih.gov/medlineplus/ency/article/003261.htm

Nail abnormalities
Web site:
http://www.nlm.nih.gov/medlineplus/ency/article/003247.htm

Nocturia
Web site:
http://www.nlm.nih.gov/medlineplus/ency/article/003141.htm

Painful menstruation
Web site:
http://www.nlm.nih.gov/medlineplus/ency/article/003150.htm

Polyuria
Web site:
http://www.nlm.nih.gov/medlineplus/ency/article/003146.htm

Stress
Web site:
http://www.nlm.nih.gov/medlineplus/ency/article/003211.htm

- **Diagnostics and Tests for Polycystic Kidney Disease**

Abdominal CT scan
Web site:
http://www.nlm.nih.gov/medlineplus/ency/article/003789.htm

Abdominal MRI
Web site:
http://www.nlm.nih.gov/medlineplus/ency/article/003796.htm

Abdominal ultrasound
Web site:
http://www.nlm.nih.gov/medlineplus/ency/article/003777.htm

ANA
Web site:
http://www.nlm.nih.gov/medlineplus/ency/article/003535.htm

Angiography
Web site:
http://www.nlm.nih.gov/medlineplus/ency/article/003327.htm

Blood pressure
Web site:
http://www.nlm.nih.gov/medlineplus/ency/article/003398.htm

BUN
Web site:
http://www.nlm.nih.gov/medlineplus/ency/article/003474.htm

CBC
Web site:
http://www.nlm.nih.gov/medlineplus/ency/article/003642.htm

Cerebral angiography
Web site:
http://www.nlm.nih.gov/medlineplus/ency/article/003799.htm

Creatinine
Web site:
http://www.nlm.nih.gov/medlineplus/ency/article/003475.htm

CT
Web site:
http://www.nlm.nih.gov/medlineplus/ency/article/003330.htm

Cyst
Web site:
http://www.nlm.nih.gov/medlineplus/ency/article/003240.htm

Cysts
Web site:
http://www.nlm.nih.gov/medlineplus/ency/article/003240.htm

Dialysis
Web site:
http://www.nlm.nih.gov/medlineplus/ency/article/003421.htm

Erythropoietin
Web site:
http://www.nlm.nih.gov/medlineplus/ency/article/003683.htm

Hematocrit
Web site:
http://www.nlm.nih.gov/medlineplus/ency/article/003646.htm

Hemoglobin
Web site:
http://www.nlm.nih.gov/medlineplus/ency/article/003645.htm

IVP
Web site:
http://www.nlm.nih.gov/medlineplus/ency/article/003782.htm

MRI
Web site:
http://www.nlm.nih.gov/medlineplus/ency/article/003335.htm

Ultrasound
Web site:
http://www.nlm.nih.gov/medlineplus/ency/article/003336.htm

Urinalysis
Web site:
http://www.nlm.nih.gov/medlineplus/ency/article/003579.htm

Urine protein
Web site:
http://www.nlm.nih.gov/medlineplus/ency/article/003580.htm

- **Surgery and Procedures for Polycystic Kidney Disease**

Kidney transplant
Web site:
http://www.nlm.nih.gov/medlineplus/ency/article/003005.htm

Nephrectomy
Web site:
http://www.nlm.nih.gov/medlineplus/ency/article/003001.htm

Renal transplant
Web site:
http://www.nlm.nih.gov/medlineplus/ency/article/003005.htm

- **Background Topics for Polycystic Kidney Disease**

Autosomal dominant
Web site:
http://www.nlm.nih.gov/medlineplus/ency/article/002049.htm

Autosomal recessive
Web site:
http://www.nlm.nih.gov/medlineplus/ency/article/002052.htm

Bleeding
Web site:
http://www.nlm.nih.gov/medlineplus/ency/article/000045.htm

Chronic
Web site:
http://www.nlm.nih.gov/medlineplus/ency/article/002312.htm

Kidney disease - support group
Web site:
http://www.nlm.nih.gov/medlineplus/ency/article/002172.htm

Renal
Web site:
http://www.nlm.nih.gov/medlineplus/ency/article/002289.htm

Support group
Web site:
http://www.nlm.nih.gov/medlineplus/ency/article/002150.htm

Systemic
Web site:
http://www.nlm.nih.gov/medlineplus/ency/article/002294.htm

Testes
Web site:
http://www.nlm.nih.gov/medlineplus/ency/article/002334.htm

Online Dictionary Directories

The following are additional online directories compiled by the National Library of Medicine, including a number of specialized medical dictionaries and glossaries:

- Medical Dictionaries: Medical & Biological (World Health Organization):
  http://www.who.int/hlt/virtuallibrary/English/diction.htm#Medical

- MEL-Michigan Electronic Library List of Online Health and Medical Dictionaries (Michigan Electronic Library):
  http://mel.lib.mi.us/health/health-dictionaries.html

- Patient Education: Glossaries (DMOZ Open Directory Project):
  http://dmoz.org/Health/Education/Patient_Education/Glossaries/

- Web of Online Dictionaries (Bucknell University):
  http://www.yourdictionary.com/diction5.html#medicine

POLYCYSTIC KIDNEY DISEASE GLOSSARY

The following is a complete glossary of terms used in this sourcebook. The definitions are derived from official public sources including the National Institutes of Health [NIH] and the European Union [EU]. After this glossary, we list a number of additional hardbound and electronic glossaries and dictionaries that you may wish to consult.

Abdomen: That portion of the body that lies between the thorax and the pelvis. [NIH]

Aberrant: Wandering or deviating from the usual or normal course. [EU]

Adenosine: A nucleoside that is composed of adenine and d-ribose. Adenosine or adenosine derivatives play many important biological roles in addition to being components of DNA and RNA. Adenosine itself is a neurotransmitter. [NIH]

Aerobic: 1. having molecular oxygen present. 2. growing, living, or occurring in the presence of molecular oxygen. 3. requiring oxygen for respiration. [EU]

Alleles: Mutually exclusive forms of the same gene, occupying the same locus on homologous chromosomes, and governing the same biochemical and developmental process. [NIH]

Aluminum: A metallic element that has the atomic number 13, atomic symbol Al, and atomic weight 26.98. [NIH]

Androgens: A class of sex hormones associated with the development and maintenance of the secondary male sex characteristics, sperm induction, and sexual differentiation. In addition to increasing virility and libido, they also increase nitrogen and water retention and stimulate skeletal growth. [NIH]

Anemia: A reduction in the number of circulating erythrocytes or in the quantity of hemoglobin. [NIH]

Aneurysm: A sac formed by the dilatation of the wall of an artery, a vein, or the heart. The chief signs of arterial aneurysm are the formation of a pulsating tumour, and often a bruit (aneurysmal bruit) heard over the swelling. Sometimes there are symptoms from pressure on contiguous parts. [EU]

Angiography: Radiography of blood vessels after injection of a contrast medium. [NIH]

Antibiotic: A chemical substance produced by a microorganism which has the capacity, in dilute solutions, to inhibit the growth of or to kill other microorganisms. Antibiotics that are sufficiently nontoxic to the host are used as chemotherapeutic agents in the treatment of infectious diseases of man, animals and plants. [EU]

Antibody: An immunoglobulin molecule that has a specific amino acid sequence by virtue of which it interacts only with the antigen that induced its synthesis in cells of the lymphoid series (especially plasma cells), or with antigen closely related to it. Antibodies are classified according to their ode of action as agglutinins, bacteriolysins, haemolysins, opsonins, precipitins, etc. [EU]

Aplasia: Lack of development of an organ or tissue, or of the cellular products from an organ or tissue. [EU]

Arteriovenous: Both arterial and venous; pertaining to or affecting an artery and a vein. [EU]

Assay: Determination of the amount of a particular constituent of a mixture, or of the biological or pharmacological potency of a drug. [EU]

Atypical: Irregular; not conformable to the type; in microbiology, applied specifically to strains of unusual type. [EU]

Bacteria: Unicellular prokaryotic microorganisms which generally possess rigid cell walls, multiply by cell division, and exhibit three principal forms: round or coccal, rodlike or bacillary, and spiral or spirochetal. [NIH]

Benign: Not malignant; not recurrent; favourable for recovery. [EU]

Bilateral: Having two sides, or pertaining to both sides. [EU]

Bile: An emulsifying agent produced in the liver and secreted into the duodenum. Its composition includes bile acids and salts, cholesterol, and electrolytes. It aids digestion of fats in the duodenum. [NIH]

Biliary: Pertaining to the bile, to the bile ducts, or to the gallbladder. [EU]

Biochemical: Relating to biochemistry; characterized by, produced by, or involving chemical reactions in living organisms. [EU]

Biopsy: The removal and examination, usually microscopic, of tissue from the living body, performed to establish precise diagnosis. [EU]

Caenorhabditis: A genus of small free-living nematodes. Two species, caenorhabditis elegans and C. briggsae are much used in studies of genetics, development, aging, muscle chemistry, and neuroanatomy. [NIH]

Calcification: The process by which organic tissue becomes hardened by a deposit of calcium salts within its substance. [EU]

Calculi: An abnormal concretion occurring mostly in the urinary and biliary tracts, usually composed of mineral salts. Also called stones. [NIH]

Capsules: Hard or soft soluble containers used for the oral administration of medicine. [NIH]

Carbohydrate: An aldehyde or ketone derivative of a polyhydric alcohol, particularly of the pentahydric and hexahydric alcohols. They are so named because the hydrogen and oxygen are usually in the proportion to form water, $(CH2O)n$. The most important carbohydrates are the starches, sugars, celluloses, and gums. They are classified into mono-, di-, tri-, poly- and heterosaccharides. [EU]

Carcinoma: A malignant new growth made up of epithelial cells tending to infiltrate the surrounding tissues and give rise to metastases. [EU]

Cardiac: Pertaining to the heart. [EU]

Cardiovascular: Pertaining to the heart and blood vessels. [EU]

Caspases: A family of intracellular cysteine endopeptidases. They play a key role in inflammation and mammalian apoptosis. They are specific for aspartic acid at the P1 position. They are divided into two classes based on the lengths of their N-terminal prodomains. Caspases-1,-2,-4,-5,-8, and -10 have long prodomains and -3,-6,-7,-9 have short prodomains. EC 3.4.22.-. [NIH]

Cerebral Angiography: Radiography of the vascular system of the brain after injection of a contrast medium. [NIH]

Chimera: An individual that contains cell populations derived from different zygotes. [NIH]

Cholecystectomy: Surgical removal of the gallbladder. [NIH]

Cholesterol: The principal sterol of all higher animals, distributed in body tissues, especially the brain and spinal cord, and in animal fats and oils. [NIH]

Chronic: Persisting over a long period of time. [EU]

Ciprofloxacin: A carboxyfluoroquinoline antimicrobial agent that is effective against a wide range of microorganisms. It has been successfully and safely used in the treatment of resistant respiratory, skin, bone, joint, gastrointestinal, urinary, and genital infections. [NIH]

Conception: The onset of pregnancy, marked by implantation of the blastocyst; the formation of a viable zygote. [EU]

Creatine: An amino acid that occurs in vertebrate tissues and in urine. In muscle tissue, creatine generally occurs as phosphocreatine. Creatine is excreted as creatinine in the urine. [NIH]

Curative: Tending to overcome disease and promote recovery. [EU]

Cyclic: Pertaining to or occurring in a cycle or cycles; the term is applied to chemical compounds that contain a ring of atoms in the nucleus. [EU]

Cysteine: A thiol-containing non-essential amino acid that is oxidized to form cystine. [NIH]

Cystinuria: An inherited abnormality of renal tubular transport of dibasic amino acids leading to massive urinary excretion of cystine, lysine, arginine, and ornithine. [NIH]

Cystitis: Inflammation of the urinary bladder. [EU]

Cytogenetics: A branch of genetics which deals with the cytological and molecular behavior of genes and chromosomes during cell division. [NIH]

Cytokines: Non-antibody proteins secreted by inflammatory leukocytes and some non-leukocytic cells, that act as intercellular mediators. They differ from classical hormones in that they are produced by a number of tissue or cell types rather than by specialized glands. They generally act locally in a paracrine or autocrine rather than endocrine manner. [NIH]

Cytoskeleton: The network of filaments, tubules, and interconnecting filamentous bridges which give shape, structure, and organization to the cytoplasm. [NIH]

Degenerative: Undergoing degeneration : tending to degenerate; having the character of or involving degeneration; causing or tending to cause degeneration. [EU]

Dementia: An acquired organic mental disorder with loss of intellectual abilities of sufficient severity to interfere with social or occupational functioning. The dysfunction is multifaceted and involves memory, behavior, personality, judgment, attention, spatial relations, language, abstract thought, and other executive functions. The intellectual decline is usually progressive, and initially spares the level of consciousness. [NIH]

Deprivation: Loss or absence of parts, organs, powers, or things that are needed. [EU]

Diarrhea: Passage of excessively liquid or excessively frequent stools. [NIH]

Drosophila: A genus of small, two-winged flies containing approximately 900 described species. These organisms are the most extensively studied of all genera from the standpoint of genetics and cytology. [NIH]

Dyes: Chemical substances that are used to stain and color other materials. The coloring may or may not be permanent. Dyes can also be used as therapeutic agents and test reagents in medicine and scientific research. [NIH]

Dysgenesis: Defective development. [EU]

Dysuria: Painful or difficult urination. [EU]

Electrophoresis: An electrochemical process in which macromolecules or colloidal particles with a net electric charge migrate in a solution under the influence of an electric current. [NIH]

Enalapril: An angiotensin-converting enzyme inhibitor that is used to treat hypertension. [NIH]

Endocrinology: A subspecialty of internal medicine concerned with the metabolism, physiology, and disorders of the endocrine system. [NIH]

Endoscopy: Visual inspection of any cavity of the body by means of an endoscope. [EU]

Endosomes: Cytoplasmic vesicles formed when coated vesicles shed their clathrin coat. Endosomes internalize macromolecules bound by receptors on the cell surface. [NIH]

Endothelium: The layer of epithelial cells that lines the cavities of the heart and of the blood and lymph vessels, and the serous cavities of the body, originating from the mesoderm. [EU]

Epidermal: Pertaining to or resembling epidermis. Called also epidermic or epidermoid. [EU]

Epinephrine: The active sympathomimetic hormone from the adrenal medulla in most species. It stimulates both the alpha- and beta- adrenergic systems, causes systemic vasoconstriction and gastrointestinal relaxation, stimulates the heart, and dilates bronchi and cerebral vessels. It is used in asthma and cardiac failure and to delay absorption of local anesthetics. [NIH]

Erythropoiesis: The production of erythrocytes. [EU]

Erythropoietin: Glycoprotein hormone, secreted chiefly by the kidney in the adult and the liver in the fetus, that acts on erythroid stem cells of the bone marrow to stimulate proliferation and differentiation. [NIH]

Exogenous: Developed or originating outside the organism, as exogenous disease. [EU]

Exons: Coding regions of messenger RNA included in the genetic transcript which survive the processing of RNA in cell nuclei to become part of a spliced messenger of structural RNA in the cytoplasm. They include joining and diversity exons of immunoglobulin genes. [NIH]

Extracellular: Outside a cell or cells. [EU]

Extrarenal: Outside of the kidney. [EU]

Fatigue: The state of weariness following a period of exertion, mental or physical, characterized by a decreased capacity for work and reduced efficiency to respond to stimuli. [NIH]

Ferritin: An iron-containing protein complex that is formed by a combination of ferric iron with the protein apoferritin. [NIH]

Fibrosis: The formation of fibrous tissue; fibroid or fibrous degeneration [EU]

Filtration: The passage of a liquid through a filter, accomplished by gravity, pressure, or vacuum (suction). [EU]

Fistula: An abnormal passage or communication, usually between two internal organs, or leading from an internal organ to the surface of the body; frequently designated according to the organs or parts with which it communicates, as anovaginal, brochocutaneous, hepatopleural, pulmonoperitoneal, rectovaginal, urethrovaginal, and the like. Such passages are frequently created experimentally for the purpose of obtaining body secretions for physiologic study. [EU]

Gastrointestinal: Pertaining to or communicating with the stomach and intestine, as a gastrointestinal fistula. [EU]

Genitourinary: Pertaining to the genital and urinary organs; urogenital; urinosexual. [EU]

Glomerular: Pertaining to or of the nature of a glomerulus, especially a renal glomerulus. [EU]

Glomerulonephritis: A variety of nephritis characterized by inflammation of the capillary loops in the glomeruli of the kidney. It occurs in acute, subacute, and chronic forms and may be secondary to haemolytic streptococcal infection. Evidence also supports possible immune or autoimmune mechanisms. [EU]

Glutamine: A non-essential amino acid present abundantly throught the body and is involved in many metabolic processes. It is synthesized from glutamic acid and ammonia. It is the principal carrier of nitrogen in the body and is an important energy source for many cells. [NIH]

Glycosuria: The presence of glucose in the urine; especially the excretion of an abnormally large amount of sugar (glucose) in the urine, i.e., more than 1 gm. in 24 hours. [EU]

Heart Murmurs: Abnormal heart sounds heard during auscultation caused by alterations in the flow of blood into a chamber, through a valve, or by a valve opening or closing abnormally. They are classified by the time of occurrence during the cardiac cycle, the duration, and the intensity of the sound on a scale of I to V. [NIH]

Hematocrit: Measurement of the volume of packed red cells in a blood specimen by centrifugation. The procedure is performed using a tube with graduated markings or with automated blood cell counters. It is used as an indicator of erythrocyte status in disease. For example, anemia shows a low hematocrit, polycythemia, high values. [NIH]

Hematology: A subspecialty of internal medicine concerned with morphology, physiology, and pathology of the blood and blood-forming tissues. [NIH]

Hematuria: Presence of blood in the urine. [NIH]

Hemorrhoids: Varicosities of the hemorrhoidal venous plexuses. [NIH]

Hepatomegaly: Enlargement of the liver. [EU]

Hernia: (he protrusion of a loop or knuckle of an organ or tissue through an abnormal opening. [EU]

Homeostasis: A tendency to stability in the normal body states (internal environment) of the organism. It is achieved by a system of control mechanisms activated by negative feedback; e.g. a high level of carbon dioxide in extracellular fluid triggers increased pulmonary ventilation, which in turn causes a decrease in carbon dioxide concentration. [EU]

Homologous: Corresponding in structure, position, origin, etc., as (a) the feathers of a bird and the scales of a fish, (b) antigen and its specific antibody, (c) allelic chromosomes. [EU]

Homozygote: An individual in which both alleles at a given locus are identical. [NIH]

Hormonal: Pertaining to or of the nature of a hormone. [EU]

Hormones: Chemical substances having a specific regulatory effect on the activity of a certain organ or organs. The term was originally applied to substances secreted by various endocrine glands and transported in the bloodstream to the target organs. It is sometimes extended to include those substances that are not produced by he endocrine glands but that have similar effects. [NIH]

Hypertelorism: Abnormal increase in the interorbital distance due to overdevelopment of the lesser wings of the sphenoid. [NIH]

Hypertension: Persistently high arterial blood pressure. Various criteria for its threshold have been suggested, ranging from 140 mm. Hg systolic and 90 mm. Hg diastolic to as high as 200 mm. Hg systolic and 110 mm. Hg diastolic. Hypertension may have no known cause (essential or idiopathic h.) or be associated with other primary diseases (secondary h.). [EU]

Induction: The act or process of inducing or causing to occur, especially the production of a specific morphogenetic effect in the developing embryo through the influence of evocators or organizers, or the production of anaesthesia or unconsciousness by use of appropriate agents. [EU]

Inflammation: A pathological process characterized by injury or destruction of tissues caused by a variety of cytologic and chemical reactions. It is usually manifested by typical signs of pain, heat, redness, swelling, and loss of function. [NIH]

Insulin: A protein hormone secreted by beta cells of the pancreas. Insulin plays a major role in the regulation of glucose metabolism, generally promoting the cellular utilization of glucose. It is also an important regulator of protein and lipid metabolism. Insulin is used as a drug to control insulin-dependent diabetes mellitus. [NIH]

Intraindividual: Being or occurring within the individual. [EU]

Invasive: 1. having the quality of invasiveness. 2. involving puncture or incision of the skin or insertion of an instrument or foreign material into the body; said of diagnostic techniques. [EU]

Iodine: A nonmetallic element of the halogen group that is represented by the atomic symbol I, atomic number 53, and atomic weight of 126.90. It is a nutritionally essential element, especially important in thyroid hormone synthesis. In solution, it has anti-infective properties and is used topically. [NIH]

Leucine: An essential branched-chain amino acid important for hemoglobin formation. [NIH]

Lipid: Any of a heterogeneous group of flats and fatlike substances characterized by being water-insoluble and being extractable by nonpolar (or fat) solvents such as alcohol, ether, chloroform, benzene, etc. All contain as a major constituent aliphatic hydrocarbons. The lipids, which are easily stored in the body, serve as a source of fuel, are an important constituent of cell structure, and serve other biological functions. Lipids may be considered to include fatty acids, neutral fats, waxes, and steroids. Compound lipids comprise the glycolipids, lipoproteins, and phospholipids. [EU]

Lithium: Lithium. An element in the alkali metals family. It has the atomic symbol Li, atomic number 3, and atomic weight 6.94. Salts of lithium are used in treating manic-depressive disorders. [NIH]

Lithotripsy: The destruction of a calculus of the kidney, ureter, bladder, or gallbladder by physical forces, including crushing with a lithotriptor through a catheter. Focused percutaneous ultrasound and focused hydraulic shock waves may be used without surgery. Lithotripsy does not include the dissolving of stones by acids or litholysis. Lithotripsy by laser is lithotripsy, laser. [NIH]

Localization: 1. the determination of the site or place of any process or lesion. 2. restriction to a circumscribed or limited area. 3. prelocalization. [EU]

Lumen: The cavity or channel within a tube or tubular organ. [EU]

Malformation: A morphologic defect resulting from an intrinsically abnormal developmental process. [EU]

Malignant: Tending to become progressively worse and to result in death. Having the properties of anaplasia, invasion, and metastasis; said of tumours. [EU]

Membrane: A thin layer of tissue which covers a surface, lines a cavity or divides a space or organ. [EU]

Metolazone: A potent, long acting diuretic useful in chronic renal disease. It also tends to lower blood pressure and increase potassium loss. [NIH]

Microgram: A unit of mass (weight) of the metric system, being one-millionth of a gram (10^{-6} gm.) or one one-thousandth of a milligram (10^{-3}

mg.). [EU]

Molecular: Of, pertaining to, or composed of molecules : a very small mass of matter. [EU]

Mutagenesis: Process of generating genetic mutations. It may occur spontaneously or be induced by mutagens. [NIH]

Myeloma: A tumour composed of cells of the type normally found in the bone marrow. [EU]

Neonatal: Pertaining to the first four weeks after birth. [EU]

Nephrology: A subspecialty of internal medicine concerned with the anatomy, physiology, and pathology of the kidney. [NIH]

Nephrons: The functional units of the kidney, consisting of the glomerulus and the attached tubule. [NIH]

Nephrosis: Descriptive histopathologic term for renal disease without an inflammatory component. [NIH]

Nephrotic: Pertaining to, resembling, or caused by nephrosis. [EU]

Neuronal: Pertaining to a neuron or neurons (= conducting cells of the nervous system). [EU]

Neurons: The basic cellular units of nervous tissue. Each neuron consists of a body, an axon, and dendrites. Their purpose is to receive, conduct, and transmit impulses in the nervous system. [NIH]

Niacin: Water-soluble vitamin of the B complex occurring in various animal and plant tissues. Required by the body for the formation of coenzymes NAD and NADP. Has pellagra-curative, vasodilating, and antilipemic properties. [NIH]

Nocturia: Excessive urination at night. [EU]

Normotensive: 1. characterized by normal tone, tension, or pressure, as by normal blood pressure. 2. a person with normal blood pressure. [EU]

Ophthalmic: Pertaining to the eye. [EU]

Orthopaedic: Pertaining to the correction of deformities of the musculoskeletal system; pertaining to orthopaedics. [EU]

Ovary: Either of the paired glands in the female that produce the female germ cells and secrete some of the female sex hormones. [NIH]

Overdose: 1. to administer an excessive dose. 2. an excessive dose. [EU]

Paclitaxel: Antineoplastic agent isolated from the bark of the Pacific yew tree, Taxus brevifolia. Paclitaxel stabilizes microtubules in their polymerized form and thus mimics the action of the proto-oncogene proteins C-MOS. [NIH]

Palliative: 1. affording relief, but not cure. 2. an alleviating medicine. [EU]

Pancreas: A mixed exocrine and endocrine gland situated transversely across the posterior abdominal wall in the epigastric and hypochondriac regions. The endocrine portion is comprised of the islets of langerhans, while the exocrine portion is a compound acinar gland that secretes digestive enzymes. [NIH]

Pancreatitis: Acute or chronic inflammation of the pancreas, which may be asymptomatic or symptomatic, and which is due to autodigestion of a pancreatic tissue by its own enzymes. It is caused most often by alcoholism or biliary tract disease; less commonly it may be associated with hyperlipaemia, hyperparathyroidism, abdominal trauma (accidental or operative injury), vasculitis, or uraemia. [EU]

Parathyroid: 1. situated beside the thyroid gland. 2. one of the parathyroid glands. 3. a sterile preparation of the water-soluble principle(s) of the parathyroid glands, ad-ministered parenterally as an antihypocalcaemic, especially in the treatment of acute hypoparathyroidism with tetany. [EU]

Patella: The flat, triangular bone situated at the anterior part of the KNEE. [NIH]

Pediatrics: A medical specialty concerned with maintaining health and providing medical care to children from birth to adolescence. [NIH]

Percutaneous: Performed through the skin, as injection of radiopacque material in radiological examination, or the removal of tissue for biopsy accomplished by a needle. [EU]

Peroxidase: A hemeprotein from leukocytes. Deficiency of this enzyme leads to a hereditary disorder coupled with disseminated moniliasis. It catalyzes the conversion of a donor and peroxide to an oxidized donor and water. EC 1.11.1.7. [NIH]

Phenotype: The outward appearance of the individual. It is the product of interactions between genes and between the genotype and the environment. This includes the killer phenotype, characteristic of yeasts. [NIH]

Phosphorylation: The introduction of a phosphoryl group into a compound through the formation of an ester bond between the compound and a phosphorus moiety. [NIH]

Poisoning: A condition or physical state produced by the ingestion, injection or inhalation of, or exposure to a deleterious agent. [NIH]

Polyuria: The passage of a large volume of urine in a given period, a characteristic of diabetes. [EU]

Postmenopausal: Occurring after the menopause. [EU]

Prevalence: The total number of cases of a given disease in a specified population at a designated time. It is differentiated from incidence, which refers to the number of new cases in the population at a given time. [NIH]

Progressive: Advancing; going forward; going from bad to worse;

increasing in scope or severity. [EU]

Protease: Proteinase (= any enzyme that catalyses the splitting of interior peptide bonds in a protein). [EU]

Proteins: Polymers of amino acids linked by peptide bonds. The specific sequence of amino acids determines the shape and function of the protein. [NIH]

Purpura: Purplish or brownish red discoloration, easily visible through the epidermis, caused by hemorrhage into the tissues. [NIH]

Pyelonephritis: Inflammation of the kidney and its pelvis, beginning in the interstitium and rapidly extending to involve the tubules, glomeruli, and blood vessels; due to bacterial infection. [EU]

Reabsorption: 1. the act or process of absorbing again, as the selective absorption by the kidneys of substances (glucose, proteins, sodium, etc.) already secreted into the renal tubules, and their return to the circulating blood. 2. resorption. [EU]

Receptor: 1. a molecular structure within a cell or on the surface characterized by (1) selective binding of a specific substance and (2) a specific physiologic effect that accompanies the binding, e.g., cell-surface receptors for peptide hormones, neurotransmitters, antigens, complement fragments, and immunoglobulins and cytoplasmic receptors for steroid hormones. 2. a sensory nerve terminal that responds to stimuli of various kinds. [EU]

Renin: An enzyme of the hydrolase class that catalyses cleavage of the leucine-leucine bond in angiotensin to generate angiotensin. 1. The enzyme is synthesized as inactive prorenin in the kidney and released into the blood in the active form in response to various metabolic stimuli. Not to be confused with rennin (chymosin). [EU]

Retrograde: 1. moving backward or against the usual direction of flow. 2. degenerating, deteriorating, or catabolic. [EU]

Riboflavin: Nutritional factor found in milk, eggs, malted barley, liver, kidney, heart, and leafy vegetables. The richest natural source is yeast. It occurs in the free form only in the retina of the eye, in whey, and in urine; its principal forms in tissues and cells are as FMN and FAD. [NIH]

Ryanodine: Insecticidal alkaloid isolated from Ryania speciosa; proposed as a myocardial depressant. [NIH]

Sclerosis: A induration, or hardening; especially hardening of a part from inflammation and in diseases of the interstitial substance. The term is used chiefly for such a hardening of the nervous system due to hyperplasia of the connective tissue or to designate hardening of the blood vessels. [EU]

Secretion: 1. the process of elaborating a specific product as a result of the activity of a gland; this activity may range from separating a specific substance of the blood to the elaboration of a new chemical substance. 2. any substance produced by secretion. [EU]

Selenium: An element with the atomic symbol Se, atomic number 34, and atomic weight 78.96. It is an essential micronutrient for mammals and other animals but is toxic in large amounts. Selenium protects intracellular structures against oxidative damage. It is an essential component of glutathione peroxidase. [NIH]

Serum: The clear portion of any body fluid; the clear fluid moistening serous membranes. 2. blood serum; the clear liquid that separates from blood on clotting. 3. immune serum; blood serum from an immunized animal used for passive immunization; an antiserum; antitoxin, or antivenin. [EU]

Somatic: 1. pertaining to or characteristic of the soma or body. 2. pertaining to the body wall in contrast to the viscera. [EU]

Species: A taxonomic category subordinate to a genus (or subgenus) and superior to a subspecies or variety, composed of individuals possessing common characters distinguishing them from other categories of individuals of the same taxonomic level. In taxonomic nomenclature, species are designated by the genus name followed by a Latin or Latinized adjective or noun. [EU]

Spectrum: A charted band of wavelengths of electromagnetic vibrations obtained by refraction and diffraction. By extension, a measurable range of activity, such as the range of bacteria affected by an antibiotic (antibacterial s.) or the complete range of manifestations of a disease. [EU]

Sterilization: 1. the complete destruction or elimination of all living microorganisms, accomplished by physical methods (dry or moist heat), chemical agents (ethylene oxide, formaldehyde, alcohol), radiation (ultraviolet, cathode), or mechanical methods (filtration). 2. any procedure by which an individual is made incapable of reproduction, as by castration, vasectomy, or salpingectomy. [EU]

Substrate: A substance upon which an enzyme acts. [EU]

Sympathectomy: The removal or interruption of some part of the sympathetic nervous system for therapeutic or research purposes. [NIH]

Thyroxine: An amino acid of the thyroid gland which exerts a stimulating effect on thyroid metabolism. [NIH]

Tomography: The recording of internal body images at a predetermined plane by means of the tomograph; called also body section roentgenography. [EU]

Toxicology: The science concerned with the detection, chemical composition, and pharmacologic action of toxic substances or poisons and the treatment and prevention of toxic manifestations. [NIH]

Transplantation: The grafting of tissues taken from the patient's own body or from another. [EU]

Tyrosine: A non-essential amino acid. In animals it is synthesized from phenylalanine. It is also the precursor of epinephrine, thyroid hormones, and melanin. [NIH]

Ultrasonography: The visualization of deep structures of the body by recording the reflections of echoes of pulses of ultrasonic waves directed into the tissues. Use of ultrasound for imaging or diagnostic purposes employs frequencies ranging from 1.6 to 10 megahertz. [NIH]

Urinalysis: Examination of urine by chemical, physical, or microscopic means. Routine urinalysis usually includes performing chemical screening tests, determining specific gravity, observing any unusual color or odor, screening for bacteriuria, and examining the sediment microscopically. [NIH]

Urinary: Pertaining to the urine; containing or secreting urine. [EU]

Urology: A surgical specialty concerned with the study, diagnosis, and treatment of diseases of the urinary tract in both sexes and the genital tract in the male. It includes the specialty of andrology which addresses both male genital diseases and male infertility. [NIH]

Ventilation: 1. in respiratory physiology, the process of exchange of air between the lungs and the ambient air. Pulmonary ventilation (usually measured in litres per minute) refers to the total exchange, whereas alveolar ventilation refers to the effective ventilation of the alveoli, in which gas exchange with the blood takes place. 2. in psychiatry, verbalization of one's emotional problems. [EU]

Zebrafish: A species of North American fishes of the family Cyprinidae. They are used in embryological studies and to study the effects of certain chemicals on development. [NIH]

General Dictionaries and Glossaries

While the above glossary is essentially complete, the dictionaries listed here cover virtually all aspects of medicine, from basic words and phrases to more advanced terms (sorted alphabetically by title; hyperlinks provide rankings, information and reviews at Amazon.com):

- **Dictionary of Medical Acronymns & Abbreviations** by Stanley Jablonski (Editor), Paperback, 4th edition (2001), Lippincott Williams & Wilkins Publishers, ISBN: 1560534605,
  http://www.amazon.com/exec/obidos/ASIN/1560534605/icongroupinterna

- **Dictionary of Medical Terms : For the Nonmedical Person (Dictionary of Medical Terms for the Nonmedical Person, Ed 4)** by Mikel A. Rothenberg, M.D, et al, Paperback - 544 pages, 4th edition (2000), Barrons Educational Series, ISBN: 0764112015,
  http://www.amazon.com/exec/obidos/ASIN/0764112015/icongroupinterna

- **A Dictionary of the History of Medicine** by A. Sebastian, CD-Rom edition (2001), CRC Press-Parthenon Publishers, ISBN: 185070368X,
  http://www.amazon.com/exec/obidos/ASIN/185070368X/icongroupinterna

- **Dorland's Illustrated Medical Dictionary (Standard Version)** by Dorland, et al, Hardcover - 2088 pages, 29th edition (2000), W B Saunders Co, ISBN: 0721662544,
  http://www.amazon.com/exec/obidos/ASIN/0721662544/icongroupinterna

- **Dorland's Electronic Medical Dictionary** by Dorland, et al, Software, 29th Book & CD-Rom edition (2000), Harcourt Health Sciences, ISBN: 0721694934,
  http://www.amazon.com/exec/obidos/ASIN/0721694934/icongroupinterna

- **Dorland's Pocket Medical Dictionary (Dorland's Pocket Medical Dictionary, 26th Ed)** Hardcover - 912 pages, 26th edition (2001), W B Saunders Co, ISBN: 0721682812,
  http://www.amazon.com/exec/obidos/ASIN/0721682812/icongroupinterna /103-4193558-7304618

- **Melloni's Illustrated Medical Dictionary (Melloni's Illustrated Medical Dictionary, 4th Ed)** by Melloni, Hardcover, 4th edition (2001), CRC Press-Parthenon Publishers, ISBN: 85070094X,
  http://www.amazon.com/exec/obidos/ASIN/85070094X/icongroupinterna

- **Stedman's Electronic Medical Dictionary Version 5.0 (CD-ROM for Windows and Macintosh, Individual)** by Stedmans, CD-ROM edition (2000), Lippincott Williams & Wilkins Publishers, ISBN: 0781726328,
  http://www.amazon.com/exec/obidos/ASIN/0781726328/icongroupinterna

- **Stedman's Medical Dictionary** by Thomas Lathrop Stedman, Hardcover - 2098 pages, 27th edition (2000), Lippincott, Williams & Wilkins, ISBN: 068340007X,
  http://www.amazon.com/exec/obidos/ASIN/068340007X/icongroupinterna

- **Tabers Cyclopedic Medical Dictionary (Thumb Index)** by Donald Venes (Editor), et al, Hardcover - 2439 pages, 19th edition (2001), F A Davis Co, ISBN: 0803606540,
  http://www.amazon.com/exec/obidos/ASIN/0803606540/icongroupinterna

INDEX

A

Abdomen 11, 15
Abdominal 26, 45, 47, 90, 204
Aberrant 63
Adenosine 42, 67, 195
Alleles 58, 69, 76, 201
Aluminum 182
Anemia...... 100, 102, 112, 179, 181, 182, 200
Aneurysm 24, 45, 195
Angiography 191
Antibiotic.................................. 26, 206
Antibody 68, 140, 198, 201
Antithrombotic...............................184
Aplasia 87
Arterial.............. 24, 25, 48, 195, 196, 201
Arteries 60
Arteriovenous...................................184
Assay...62
Atypical 60

B

Bacteria.........................26, 146, 206
Benign..87
Bilateral 77, 138
Bile....................................28, 99, 196
Biliary 52, 67, 85, 90, 196, 204
Biochemical 54, 61, 67, 195
Biopsy 70, 204

C

Calcification 86
Calculi 47
Capsules 149
Carbohydrate...........................45, 148
Carcinoma 47, 87
Cardiac..........21, 45, 47, 85, 86, 199, 200
Cardiovascular...........................86, 183
Caspases 55
Cholecystectomy..............................93
Cholesterol 146, 148
Chronic.....25, 28, 44, 77, 85, 90, 92, 100, 136, 137, 138, 144, 152, 167, 180, 200, 202, 204
Conception 12, 16
Creatine.................................. 118, 197
Curative.........................53, 156, 203
Cyclic..42, 57
Cysteine 55
Cystinuria 87, 88
Cystitis 87
Cytogenetics....................................75
Cytokines 184

Cytoskeleton................................. 50, 66

D

Degenerative 147
Deprivation 59
Diarrhea 146
Drosophila...60
Dyes 13
Dysgenesis.......................................85

E

Electrophoresis.................................75
Enalapril...............................138, 153
Endoscopy 43
Endosomes 50
Epidermal 42, 63
Epinephrine 182
Erythropoiesis................................. 137
Erythropoietin 44, 100, 179, 180
Exogenous 64, 68, 199
Extracellular......41, 42, 44, 45, 50, 61, 68, 201
Extrarenal.............. 41, 44, 52, 59, 85, 86

F

Fatigue 21, 100
Ferritin 182
Fibrosis 28, 52, 63, 85, 87, 99
Filtration 40, 48, 62, 88, 106, 206
Fistula 200

G

Gastrointestinal...... 47, 86, 129, 183, 197, 199, 200
Glomerular 40, 48, 62, 88
Glomerulonephritis....17, 88, 92, 106, 107
Glutamine...................................... 118
Glycosuria 87

H

Hematocrit.................100, 102, 180, 200
Hematology 10
Hematuria 17, 43, 44, 46, 47, 86, 87
Hemorrhoids 15
Hepatic............28, 45, 56, 63, 87, 99, 152
Homeostasis....................................50
Homologous 59, 61, 67, 195
Hormonal 152
Hormones 16, 70, 89, 90, 99, 195, 198, 203, 205
Hypertension 40, 41, 42, 44, 46, 47, 52, 58, 85, 86, 88, 92, 99, 106, 143, 152, 198

I

Induction 64, 89, 195
Infantile 15, 22

Inflammation 25, 67, 71, 90, 106, 197, 200, 204, 205
Inguinal 85
Insulin 89, 201
Interstitial...............................71, 87, 205
Intraindividual..................................100

L
Leucine 41, 51, 70, 205
Lipid 60, 62, 89, 151, 201
Lithium 154, 156, 202
Lithotripsy 43
Localization................................. 43, 55
Lumen...53

M
Malformation 99
Malignant....................... 67, 84, 196, 197
Medullary...87
Membrane ..41, 42, 43, 45, 48, 50, 55, 60, 64, 151
Metolazone.....................................137
Molecular....10, 18, 41, 42, 46, 49, 52, 56, 57, 59, 62, 70, 86, 101, 104, 109, 110, 118, 141, 195, 198, 205
Mutagenesis 60, 62
Myeloma...87

N
Neonatal..40
Nephrons 12
Nephropathy 87, 88, 138
Nephrosis.........................90, 106, 203
Nephrotic...88
Neuronal...50
Neurons.................................... 49, 203
Niacin...146
Normotensive 46, 152

O
Overdose...147

P
Paclitaxel...141
Palliative..52
Pancreas 15, 60, 84, 89, 90, 201, 204
Patella...87
Percutaneous.......................43, 69, 202
Peroxidase 61
Phenotype 46, 51, 54, 59, 70, 204
Phosphorylation 51
Poisoning 182
Postmenopausal 180, 181
Prenatal...............................22, 76, 86
Prevalence 80, 183
Progressive 28, 48, 52, 60, 65, 74, 76, 86, 89, 99, 153, 183, 198

Prostatitis 87
Proteins 41, 43, 45, 50, 54, 55, 59, 60, 144, 146, 148, 198, 205
Pulmonary 68, 99, 201
Purpura 87
Pyelonephritis 106

R
Reabsorption 141
Receptor ...45, 50, 55, 57, 60, 61, 63, 140
Renin...44
Retrograde 43
Riboflavin 146
Ryanodine..55

S
Sclerosis 45, 75, 112
Secretion 44, 53, 71, 206
Selenium 61, 148
Serum ... 43, 48, 55, 59, 71, 141, 181, 206
Somatic...................................44, 58, 61
Species 61, 67, 68, 71, 196, 198, 199, 206, 207
Spectrum...10
Splenomegaly..................................93
Sterilization 183
Substrate...51
Sympathectomy 93

T
Testicular 45
Thermoregulation.............................146
Thoracic..45
Thyroxine 148
Tomography 13, 21, 22
Toxicologic 152
Toxicology 10, 105
Transplantation 11, 15, 16, 18, 46, 47, 54, 75, 80, 84, 86, 92, 99, 106, 137, 181, 183
Tyrosine 51

U
Ultrasonography 22, 40
Urinalysis 207
Urinary . 14, 15, 16, 17, 21, 26, 44, 47, 48, 67, 89, 106, 129, 196, 197, 198, 200, 207
Urology 10

V
Vascular............. 21, 47, 82, 86, 152, 197
Veins..15
Ventilation 68, 99, 102, 201, 207

Z
Zebrafish...62

Printed in the United States
24787LVS00001B/31

9 780597 832277